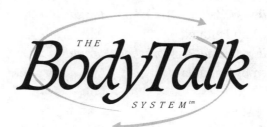

COMMUNICATE/SYNCHRONIZE/BALANCE

The BodyTalk System™

*The missing link
to optimum health.*

by John Veltheim

PUBLISHED BY PARAMA

Also by John Veltheim
 Acupuncture—How it Works, and How it Can Help You
 Published by Hill of Content, Melbourne, Australia
 BodyTalk, Module 1—Workshop Manual
 Published by PaRama
 BodyTalk, Module 2—Workshop Manual
 Published by PaRama

By John & Esther Veltheim
 Reiki: The Science, Metaphysics, and Philosophy
 Published by PaRama

First published in September 1999
Second printing in November 1999
by
PaRama INC.
5500 Bee Ridge Drive, #103
Sarasota, FL 34233, USA

ISBN 0-9645944-9-8

Printed in the USA

e-mail: parama@home.com
Web site: www.parama.com
IBA Web site: www.bodytalksystem.com

Book and Cover Design by Colleen Clinton

Dedicated to my wife
Esther
She has become the spark behind BodyTalk...
and the mentor of its development.

Contents

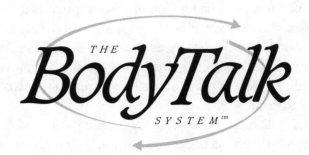

Introduction

GARY

Gary had severe glandular fever, Epstein-Barr virus, when he was 39 years old. Although he recovered from the acute stage of the illness, he was left with a chronic virus. This Chronic Fatigue Syndrome left Gary extremely tired. He also had aching muscles, headaches, muscle cramps, an inability to exercise or do physical work, and a chronic temperature. Doctors even told him he could end up in a wheelchair, since the virus was still present in his blood after several years.

Conventional medicine offered nothing, so he had extensive treatments with herbal and homeopathic remedies, chiropractic, acupuncture, and Reiki. After six years there was no improvement and Gary still suffered with pain, headaches, depression, and fatigue on a daily basis.

After his second BodyTalk treatment, Gary had an immune reaction that lasted three days. His temperature rose to 103°F and he experienced flu-like symptoms. A few days later though he was feeling great. All symptoms of the Chronic Fatigue Syndrome had disappeared. The next week Gary had blood tests that verified the virus had gone. All that was left were the signs of increased antigen activity; signifying that his immune system had finally beaten the virus.

CAROL

Carol arrived at my clinic justifiably distressed. She had been told by a medical specialist that she had only a few days to live and there was no help they could offer her. Carol had a form of vasculitis that had been treated with massive doses of cortisone without results. She had parasites throughout the vascular system that were destroying the walls of the blood vessels, causing them to hemorrhage. While there was evidence of this hemorrhaging under her skin, the main problem was the internal hemorrhaging: it was causing her to slowly bleed to death.

The BodyTalk treatment enabled her immune system to specifically target the parasite problem and its underlying causes. Within nine hours all the parasites and had been destroyed by her immune system; she fully recovered within a few days. Carol is now a BodyTalk practitioner.

JENNY

Jenny had a skiing accident and dislocated her right shoulder. Because she had previously been treated successfully for sports injuries with BodyTalk, she insisted on coming to me rather than to the hospital. By the time she got to my office two hours had passed since the accident and inflammation had set in, making the job of relocating the shoulder very difficult. We gently held the shoulder and the hip on the opposite side to establish a reciprocal relationship and tapped the head and sternum. What followed was truly amazing: within a few minutes there was an active reduction in pain followed by a series of contractions and relaxations of the various muscles around the shoulder. To our amazement the shoulder was then relatively painlessly pulled back into place *by the muscles*. Within 15 minutes Jenny had full range of motion in her shoulder and the next day had little evidence of the problem.

ANN

Ann suffered from an extreme fear of spiders. The phobia was so bad that when she saw a spider she immediately started projectile vomiting. Needless to say this was a serious problem that curtailed her social life. She was afraid to go anywhere, fearing that a spider would appear and cause her great embarrassment.

The BodyTalk treatment for arachnophobia—and most fears and phobias—is simple: disassociate the emotional traumatic memory relating to the

---

phobia from normal brain activity. It took only one treatment to completely eliminate the phobia and give Ann her life back.

PAM

Pam, 62 years old, fell down the stairs and was unable to turn her head to the left or tilt it backwards for two years despite extensive therapy from a variety of practitioners. She was told that the combination of arthritis and age would stop her from ever regaining her mobility.

After ten minutes of BodyTalk treatment the range of motion in her neck had improved 70 percent. Two more treatments restored full range of motion and Pam is now pain free.

JOHN

Seven-year-old John caught the flu that was going around his school. He woke up with a temperature, sore throat, painful chest, cough, and headache. His mother had been taught the simple BodyTalk treatment for treating infections and viruses (covered in this book) and immediately treated John. No medication was given. She kept him home and noticed that for the next few hours his temperature increased quite rapidly and, at first, his symptoms appeared to get worse. By the afternoon his temperature and symptoms decreased just as rapidly as they had appeared. John woke up the next morning symptom free and went to school. He couldn't help noting that his other friends with the same flu were ill for at least a week.

LYNN

Lynn's holiday in Mexico turned into a nightmare. She arrived home riddled with parasites that caused explosive diarrhea, stomach cramps, vomiting and severe distress. She immediately went to her next door neighbor for a BodyTalk treatment. The treatment activated Lynn's immune system to kill the parasites and within two days she was back to normal.

ALICE

Alice had never recovered from the shock and grief associated with the sudden death of her husband from a heart attack. She was engulfed in a depression so deep she could not shake it off, no matter how hard she tried to get involved in life. The depression had weakened her immune system and she found herself catching everything that went around. She was constantly going to the doctor for antibiotics and feeling weak and tired.

BodyTalk reestablished all the communication systems that had been shut down through the shock of her husband's death. Her body was finally able to process the grief, and reestablish the endocrine and immune systems to normalcy. Alice's recovery was spectacular. Within one week she felt alive and vital and was able to look forward to the coming years.

Although the previous cases are different, and cover a wide variety of human ailments, they were all treated simply and effectively; using BodyTalk to reestablish communication between all the body parts.

No medications were given, no therapies applied, no diagnosis was made, and, in every case, the patient's own body dictated what was treated, in what order, and in what frequency. This is the wonder of BodyTalk and on the following pages we are going to explore this magic.

BodyTalk is what happens when you combine the wisdom of advanced yoga and advaita philosophy, the insights of modern physics and mathematics, the energy dynamics of acupuncture, the clinical findings of Applied Kinesiology, and Western medical expertise.

As a result of this synthesis of knowledge, both ancient and modern, BodyTalk has the potential to revolutionize the treatment protocol of all alternative and orthodox healing modalities.

The BodyTalk System™ can be applied across the board in conjunction with all other therapies, as well as being a stand-alone treatment modality. Its major assets are simplicity, safety, and the speed of its results. It works as effectively on animals as it does on people and even has application in the treatment of plants.

You cannot hurt someone with BodyTalk. If you perform a technique incorrectly, it simply means there will be no result or change. It will not make the situation worse.

By explaining the principles and philosophy behind The BodyTalk System™, and teaching you many of the simple BodyTalk techniques, I hope to show you that BodyTalk represents a new paradigm for health care in the 21st century. It is a non-invasive and simple system that engenders a total respect for the innate wisdom found within each and every living entity. When this wisdom is tapped into and utilized, miracles of healing can occur.

Basic Premises of BodyTalk

BODY WISDOM

1. The body has an innate wisdom which, when allowed, can heal the body at all levels.
2. This innate wisdom can even tell us what is wrong with the body, what needs to be treated, and in what order.
3. The key element in maintaining health in the body is the reestablishment of communication between all the systems and parts of the body. In this way, the body can synchronize its activities, heal, and adapt to the stresses of life.
4. The most important consideration in the healing process is the sequence in which the body heals the systems. One of the main factors that slows down the healing process is the superimposition of the bias and agenda of the practitioner.
5. The more we respect the body's inate wisdom (higher self, witness, source, whatever you wish to call it), the more it instructs us and the more powerful it becomes.

TREATMENT PRINCIPLES

1. ASKING THE BODY.

The body can be asked what is wrong through muscle testing (biofeedback). By establishing a *yes/no* communication system, the body can instruct us as to its needs once we learn the protocol for systematically covering the entire bodymind complex.

2. LINKING.

Linking is the key to the new paradigm of treatment. The practitioner must ask the body what parts need to be linked in order to reestablish good communication and facilitate healing.

3. THE TAPPING PROCESS.

The tapping process is used on the head and sternum (heart) to facilitate the linkage and store it.

4. EXAGGERATED BREATHING.

Exaggerated breathing is often used to help the body locate and target the corrections.

Innate Wisdom

The body has an innate wisdom which, when allowed, can heal the body at all levels.

TO THOSE OF YOU WHO HAVE BEEN INVESTIGATING alternative medicine this statement seems obvious. However, I challenge you to really think about what the statement means. I feel we often neglect to recognize how powerfully we can tap into the innate wisdom of the body.

We all know that the body has a built-in mechanism that initiates the healing process in normal day-to-day activity. If we cut ourselves, the body immediately sets up a process to start healing the wound. This occurs at all levels—physical, emotional, and mental. Although this process is obvious to all of us, it is my experience that most systems of healing do not give full credence to how wonderful the human mechanism really is—or to its potential. They also fail to recognize its potential.

We are quick to play God, making our own personal diagnosis and telling our body how to heal itself based on our (perceived) superior knowledge of the healing process. Granted, you may say you only step in when your body is

13

failing to do its job. The body, however, is only failing in its job because its communications systems have been severely compromised through the stresses of life and the interference superimposed upon it. Once you reestablish a good communication system between the various parts of the body, the body can—and will—heal, except in extreme emergency situations.

The trouble is that up to now the focus has not been on communication. The focus has been on *repairing the parts that appear to be problems and hoping the body can then get those parts to synchronize.* The new paradigm states that the focus should be on restoring the synchronization and the body will repair its own parts rapidly. The resultant dynamic energy configuration will allow the parts to quickly return to normal synchronized activity within the bodymind complex and its environment.

Mankind has blown its knowledge of the workings of the body out of proportion. Since we have learned a great deal about the physiological processes of the body, we tend to think we can play God with this knowledge. In recent years it has become increasingly obvious that our knowledge about the workings of the body is still at a kindergarten level. You may point to many textbooks that show an enormous wealth of knowledge, puffing your chest up with pride at the immense amount of information we have accumulated about the body, but that is like looking at an encyclopedia and saying it has all the knowledge of the world contained in it. That knowledge is just a drop in the ocean.

Everyday we receive more and more evidence of just how intricate a system the bodymind complex is. The immense interrelationships between the components of the body at the physical level, i.e. energy systems, environmental factors, and mental and emotional components, create a complex symphony of relationships of which we are only beginning to scratch the surface. The joke is we think we have the knowledge to tell the body how to do its job when it has been doing that job successfully for millions of years. How arrogant we are!

There are times, you might say, when the body fails to do that job and needs help. True, but the type of help it has been getting is not necessarily what it really wants—or needs—for most problems.

The real problem facing the body is in the way our life styles, culture, and technology have interfered with the natural processes; compromising the com-

14

munication networks that enable it to coordinate the billions of synchronized activities per second necessary to maintain optimum health.

The BodyTalk paradigm for the future of medicine is one where we once again start respecting the awesome innate knowledge of the body and learn to utilize that knowledge by working with it, rather than imposing our pathetic, childish knowledge upon it.

CHAPTER

3

Directions from the Higher Self

The body's innate wisdom can even tell us what is wrong with it, what needs to be treated, and in what order.

THROUGHOUT HISTORY MANKIND HAS BEEN AWARE OF how powerful intuition can be. Most people, unfortunately, have found the art of intuition has been lost because of the doubts wrought by intellectual criticism and cynicism. We have spent so much time examining the world, dividing it up into parts, and analyzing it from an intellectual, scientific perspective, we have lost touch—and confidence—in our own innate wisdom. There seems to be only a small percentage of the population who are fortunate enough to have been raised by parents who encouraged creative, right-brain, intuitive awareness.

Just because we have lost touch with awareness doesn't mean it is gone. The fact that we heal in normal circumstances shows our innate wisdom is still there doing its job, given the circumstances limiting its function.

By acknowledging this innate wisdom, The BodyTalk System™ can communicate with that wisdom to ask what is *really* wrong with the body, what needs to be treated, and, most importantly, in what order.

Another consideration that is important when treating a patient is to recognize that every person is unique. They each have different genetic makeup, personalities, belief systems, and environmental influences.

This all means they will each have different bodily functions and balances. When we are treating someone, the danger lies in trying to influence their health to conform to our judgement of what is normal.

Society loves to take surveys and assess the behavior and health of the majority. Practitioners can often fall into the trap of subconsciously accepting those parameters. This means that they often try to correct the patient's bodymind balance to fit within those common parameters rather than the individual patterns of the unique bodymind they are treating. This leads to creating an artificial balance that can be harmful, in the long run, to the patient.

Only the innate wisdom of the body knows the right balance for that particular bodymind. Therefore, nothing should be treated without the 'blessing' of the innate wisdom. I am certain that, in the future, society will start to realize it has allowed science—and egotistical minds—to tamper with nature far too much. We are beginning to see this in environmental matters; where the balance of the environment was drastically altered because we didn't understand as much of earth's delicate balance as we thought we did.

This same scenario is happening with the human body. We are tampering with it long before we have an intimate knowledge of how it works. Don't kid yourself, we may know a lot, but that knowledge is only at kindergarten level compared to what is still there for discovery. The mere fact that BodyTalk works is already a challenge to the 'accepted' knowledge of physiology. Most times, the studies done to determine harmful side effects are short term. Any long term studies are largely disregarded because there are too many parameters to consider.

It is imperative that we seriously consider the paradigm I am presenting in this book before we find that we have done irreversible damage to the genetic structure of the human form. There is a very real scenario of the human race becoming extinct through genetic destruction in much the same way as some species of animals have been wiped out.

It is also important to let a patient know that they have this unique

18

bodymind and an innate intelligence to know what is right for them. Many patients come in with an agenda for their treatment. They have listened to the stories of others and what 'most people' do, believing that to be healthy they must have that same treatment to achieve wellness. These patients need to be counseled about accepting their own true nature based on their genetic and environmental background. Once they realize that you are asking their body what is, uniquely, right for them, they will begin the process of individuation that will enable them to find the right balance for their life: physically, emotionally, mentally, and spiritually.

CHAPTER

4

Reestablishing Communication

The key element in maintaining health in the body is reestablishment of communication between all systems and parts of the body.

IN THE LAST FEW CENTURIES THERE HAVE BEEN TWO major trends in scientific thought. The Cartesian model, established in the last two centuries, was based on the premise that the world was like a big clock. Descartes theorized that all we had to do was dissect and examine all its parts thoroughly in order to solve the mysteries of existence. This model sounded great and science launched into the study of mathematics and science with great enthusiasm. It was a huge boost to the egos of the people involved.

Then, at the turn-of-the-century, physicists and mathematicians discovered that Descartes' theory was somewhat simplistic. The laws of relativity and quantum mechanics quickly showed scientists that the model of the clock was not valid except in relative conditions. So even though quantum mechanics proved Descartes' theory invalid some ninety years ago, there is still a primitive tendency to approach medicine, and the treatment of the body, along the archaic Cartesian lines of reasoning. This tendency still occurs because it appeals to our natural inclination to use simple logic to explain the world despite all evidence to the contrary. That is, that there are no logical or ultimate explanations.

By tracing the discoveries of quantum mechanics through to the present time, we see the evolution of the holographic paradigm. Quantum mechanics views the world as being in constant dynamic interaction at all levels; nothing existing in, and of, itself. Everything, from this perspective, exists only as part of a dynamic system, with each part reflecting the whole.

Bells theorem emphasizes that *"no theory of reality compatible with quantum theory can require specially separated events to be separate."* In other words, all distant events are constantly interconnected and interdependent. This implies that each and every electron must know exactly what every other electron in the universe is doing in order to understand what it, itself, has to do at any given moment. This further implies that every atom in the universe is constantly "in touch" with "all that is." This universality (or interconnectedness) of substance corresponds to the concept of a consciousness that is cognizant of everything—collectively and individually. This paradigm postulates that every microscopic part of our body knows exactly what every other part is doing and is responding accordingly. The innate wisdom of the individual body is therefore connected to the wisdom of *totality as a whole*. By utilizing this wisdom, we are tapping into universal consciousness.

In his book, *The Web of Life*, physicist Fritjof Capra summarizes the view of the famous quantum physicist Geoffrey Chew who developed the 'bootstrap' theory to explain the observed phenomena of sub-atomic particles:

> *The 'bootstrap' philosophy declares that we must abandon the idea of fundamental building blocks of matter. There are no fundamental entities whatsoever—no fundamental constants, laws, or equations. The material universe is seen as a dynamic web of interrelated events. None of the properties of any part of this web is fundamental. They all follow from the properties of other parts, and the overall consistency of their interrelations determines the structure of the entire web.*

This further reinforces the concept of synchronicity. Concordant with this concept is the conclusion that everything within the body is in a dynamic,

22

synchronized, interactive, and totally inter/intra-dependant state.

This concept is called Dynamic Systems Theory. Through the Dynamic Systems Theory, all branches of alternative medicine have the potential of developing a solid, theoretical framework for working with the body as an energy system. Dynamic Systems Theory also goes a long way in explaining the nuances of the mindbody relationship particularly in relation to energy healing. The diverse and controversial findings and observations of the human energy system are finally explainable in relative terms.

The integration of the concepts of energy that come from physics, with the concept of a dynamic biological system, emphasize *dynamic, interactive, communicative, conscious relationships within systems and between systems.* This is important when we study:

• The relationship of the brain to the rest of the body;
• The relationship of the heart to the rest of the body, and
• All the other combinations within the body.

Some branches of physics have had a traditional tendency to study mindbody systems as if they are 'closed' structures with simple linear relationships to other structures. This is very evident in classical medicine. The Dynamic Systems Theory approach sees them as they really are: dynamic, interactive, complex information processors that develop their own systems of memory, consciousness and innate wisdom (awareness). This approach assumes that the systems are spontaneously fluctuating (an assumption consistent with quantum mechanics); and are always 'open' systems interacting with all the other systems around them to varying degrees over time. This also implies that systems within the body are a consistently interacting and evolving consciousness with all the systems within the environment (clothes, other living systems, climate, and so on).

Despite existing scientific and mathematical knowledge, the medical model has continued to disregard the important lessons learned from the Dynamic Systems Theory. Allopathic and alternative medical systems have continued to try and break the body down into parts. Consequently, the workings of the body continue to be investigated by means of this simplistic linear model. Traditional medicine has tended to limit its analysis of the body to that which is tangible and can be readily dissected or examined under a microscope. Theoretically it tries to relate to the body in the form of simple chemical interactions.

This is despite the fact that science has clearly demonstrated the body is simple energy interacting with energy in a multitude of forms. The physical, tangible aspect is only one small part of a total dynamic interactive process interacting with itself and its environment.

Medicine can no longer afford to labor under an antiquated system of looking at the world. In the 21st century it must have the courage to look seriously at what science has been saying for a hundred years and accept that a new paradigm must evolve in the treatment of disease. This paradigm would be based on recognition of the living dynamic interrelationships within the body. There would be recognition that all interrelationships are being synchronized and coordinated by an innate wisdom infinitely greater in intelligence than even the most sophisticated computers.

It would be primitive and counterproductive to treat the body through diagnosis and intervention. The exception would be in emergencies where the natural process is too damaged to repair itself. The key will be in cooperating with the innate wisdom of consciousness to restore the vital interrelationships by linking the critical components that have lost their lines of communication. This will then enable the necessary synchronicity of bodymind activities for restoration of dynamic health relative to the individual needs of that particular system.

An analogy can be made with a symphony orchestra. You can have seventy finely tuned instruments in a symphony orchestra, each capable of making a beautiful sound, but if you do not have a conductor to synchronize the playing of the instruments the end result will be a noise, not a symphony. The parts of the body are like the parts of that symphony orchestra. If they are synchronized by the innate wisdom within the body, then there will be a symphony of health. *Poor health occurs when the communication systems and energy linkages necessary for innate wisdom to function optimally are compromised.* This is where BodyTalk comes in. In the The BodyTalk System™ we ask the body what it requires to reestablish all the communication systems necessary for it to do its job.

The key element here is in realizing that treatment of individual body parts will not necessarily lead to good health. Most systems of medicine concentrate on treating individual parts or systems—and we are not talking about only traditional medicine. Everyone knows the folly of having a patient go to a heart specialist for the heart, a kidney specialist for the kidneys, and a urologist for the bladder. In the meantime, none of the doctors know about any of the other doctors treating that same patient. Each doctor is only concentrating on his own speciality, often ignoring the dynamic interrelationships between all the organs and the importance of synchronicity in their activities.

I have also found that alternative medicine is very guilty of doing exactly the same thing. Patients receive treatment from several practitioners at the same time and none of them are coordinating their efforts. Although alternative medical practitioners pay lip service to being holistic in their approach, the fact remains that the majority are still only focusing on individual systems. They may treat the meridians, the chakras, and the digestive system in the form of diet, the spine, the muscular system, the emotions, and so on; but this is not a truly holistic approach since they are still treating individual systems, much the same as a heart specialist treats just the heart and cardiovascular system. All alternative medicine is doing is looking at isolated sets of frequencies within the bodymind complex.

In the new paradigm presented in this book, I propose that in the future we must look at linking the entire spectrum of systems (physical and energic) and recognizing each individual system as part of a whole.

The actual BodyTalk treatment protocol allows for this. Besides being a protocol for a nearly complete system in its own right, the protocol provides a link between all the systems. It forms a bridge between physical medicine and energy medicine and everything in between. Each modality slots into the over-all protocol and the bodymind's innate wisdom will readily take advantage of the particular system in which the practitioner has expertise.

The Sequence of Healing

The most important consideration in the healing process is the sequence in which the body heals the systems.

THE CONCEPT OF IN WHAT ORDER TO TREAT IS NOT something readily thought about in most systems of health care. In my many years of being in practice, running colleges, and training practitioners, I have seen that the difference between the top practitioners and the others is often found in:

1) Their decision as to what to treat and, more importantly;

2) Knowing in what order to treat specific conditions.

For most practitioners, the easy part of treatment is to come up with a list of symptoms and a subsequent diagnosis. The key element in good therapy is to know in which order to treat each of the conditions and in which order to evoke repair of the organs, endocrines, or body parts. Very often practitioners designate the course their treatment takes by relying on their own fixed agenda or bias created from their training background.

In my observations of acupuncturists, I saw the spleen-oriented acupuncturist, one who always found a weak spleen that needed to be treated first. This was usually because she had a personal background of spleen disorders. Other practitioners may be kidney practitioners who tend to treat the kidney complex first because of their own background of weak kidneys. Naturopaths are quick to find toxic livers in most patients in our society and are very quick to prescribe diets and herbs designed to detoxify the liver. Others want patients to fast and then give them colonic irrigations to clean out the stomach and intestines.

The vital fact most people fail to recognize is that the body will respond best if you *treat all the conditions in exactly the right sequence necessary to reestablish a dynamic system.* Very often the body does not want the liver detoxified until the small intestine is treated or until the adrenals are tonified or the thyroid is balanced to the function of the pituitary gland, etc.

When the practitioner prescribes a liver cleanse and it is not appropriate for the body at that particular time, the patient will often experience a worsening of the symptoms. This is often described as a healing crisis. Indeed, sometimes it is a valid healing crisis, but other times it is simply bad management. The body is not prepared to clean the liver out until the other system relationships are established first. If this protocol is not recognized, the body will have an adverse reaction to the liver cleanse. This will, paradoxically, slow down healing or overstress the entire system to the point that it cannot heal.

This concept applies to all modalities of health care. It would be preferable that, before a surgeon operates, she asks the body what needs to be done *before the operation* in order for it to take full advantage of that operation. Very often the reason the patient has trouble recovering is because the rest of the dynamic system of the bodymind had not been correctly prepared to take full advantage of the ramifications of the operation.

When a chiropractor is adjusting the spine there are often subluxations apparent in the spine. The chiropractor should be aware that the body will respond far better if the adjustments are performed in the exact sequence the body wants. For example, sometimes the body prefers that the pelvis and sacroiliac joints be stabilized first. On other occasions it may want the cervical vertebrae or a mid-dorsal vertebra stabilized first. At other times it may be preferable to use other methods such as myofacial release or dietary supplements first.

I have found that, in medicine, the actual sequence in which drugs are taken by the patient can have critical ramifications. BodyTalk can be used to quickly establish the right sequence, dosage, and combinations of drugs, supplements, herbs, or homeopathics that are best for the individual patient.

We must remember that the body is a total, holistic, interrelated system that involves billions of interrelationships and linkages. Some of those linkages can be quite obscure and involve a dynamic that is way beyond the comprehension of a practitioner. The BodyTalk System™ recognizes this dynamic and therefore follows the protocol that:

- No treatment is given until the body asks for it.
- The treatments are given in the exact sequence asked for by the body, in the exact number of treatments asked for by the body.

For example, a patient may come in with a back problem and the BodyTalk protocol will establish that the body wants the stomach, psoas muscle, and rib cage balanced before any treatment is given on the back. The body may not even allow the back to be treated on the first visit. Instead, it wants the original balancing to have time to work before the balancing of the back occurs. It will even tell the practitioner the exact day to bring the patient back for further treatment. Time and again I have seen the patient's symptoms disappear, even though I had not directly treated the location of the discomfort.

In many cases the symptoms are not located near the cause of the disease. The so-called disease is merely the tip of an iceberg. The disease is a collection of symptoms to which we give a fancy name. The true cause underlying the disease is usually a combination of many different factors. Most diseases have many ingredients behind them including such things as dietary indiscretions, stress factors, emotional imbalance, environmental toxins, and physical injuries. There are also a score of other factors that we are not usually aware of, such as environmental relationship problems between the patient's energy field and the energy fields of people and objects within the normal daily environment of the patient.

A practitioner cannot hope to fully understand the enormous complexity of all these relationships or to work out an optimal formula to reestablish dynamic healthy synchronicity of all these factors. It is only the innate wisdom of the body that is capable of such a prodigious task. For effective healing at the deepest level we must acknowledge this enormous tool at our disposal, listen to it, and follow its instructions.

I am convinced that this concept of treatment is one of the most important breakthroughs in modern health care. The BodyTalk System™ will form the backbone of cutting edge health care early in the new millennium.

Respecting the Innate Wisdom

The more we respect the body's innate wisdom, the more it instructs us and the more powerful it becomes.

I AM USING THE TERM 'INNATE WISDOM' BECAUSE IT probably has fewer connotations in meaning. We could use the terms higher self, witness, source, innate intelligence, awareness, etc., according to cultural or academic background. What I am, in fact, referring to is that innate consciousness in the body we observe every day of our lives. It is the force that keeps the system going, healing, harmonizing, and attempting to create a healthy situation. I refer to it later in this book as a state of awareness. I will demonstrate that it appears to be contained in the heart complex in the chest.

We talk of certain people being more aware than others. Some have an innate tendency to trust their intuition more, heal faster, and have an intuitive understanding of what is best for their body. Those people who do not seem to have as great an awareness are often people who come from a background that has discouraged this inner communication with the body. It is very sad this has happened; and so many have lost contact with that very real part of themselves.

I have found that when a patient undergoes a series of BodyTalk treatments, their level of the awareness rises quickly. When their innate wisdom is consulted directly, as it is with The BodyTalk System™, that awareness tends to rise to the occasion and supply the needed feedback. At some level, the BodyTalk balancing of the system helps to put the patient back into that natural state of awareness, thereby making them more responsive to treatment in future sessions. The body seems to learn the language of communication at this deep level with the practitioner. This enables the body to make more sophisticated links for healing and balancing the system faster.

One of the most common side effects of a BodyTalk treatment is that patients often notice an increased state of well being and general harmony with their body and mind. This well being is subjective in nature, but very real to the patient. Once the patient starts experiencing this stronger harmonious relationship with their body, the innate wisdom is better able to maintain optimum health in the future.

I have noticed that patients I treated a year ago who have returned for a different health problem, respond much faster the second time around. The original BodyTalk sessions helped reestablish the relationship with an awareness that is still there a year later.

CHAPTER

7

Treatment Principles

Muscle Testing: Asking the Body

The body can be asked what is wrong through muscle testing (bio-feedback). BY ESTABLISHING A *YES/NO* COMMUNICATION SYSTEM, the body can instruct us as to its needs once we learn the protocol for systematically covering the entire bodymind complex.

There are many ways to obtain biofeedback from the body. In The BodyTalk System™ we primarily utilize muscle testing to achieve that end. When we first start developing our ability to muscle test, we rely on testing for variations in muscle strength; although, ultimately, we will not be using muscle strength as such. We will be training the patient to respond to questions with a yes or no answer; the muscle appears weak for a *yes* answer and strong for a *no* answer.

The strength of our muscles is dependent on many factors. We are aware we can be stronger on some days and weaker on others. We know that our moods and emotional state can greatly affect the strength of our muscles. The muscles go a long way toward reflecting our state of health.

Applied Kinesiology has shown us that if we test any muscle in our body, and then 'challenge' the body in a way that affects the body, the muscle, when retested, will be weaker for a short period of time. This change lasts for a short time.

With The BodyTalk System™ we take advantage of that observed phenomena. When we touch trigger points on the body and ask if there is a problem, the body will answer '*yes*' by letting the muscle appear weak. Any muscle in the body can be used. We tend to use the shoulder muscles for convenience and because they don't tire easily.

After linking the trigger points with a BodyTalk treatment, we ask once more if there is a problem. This time the body will answer '*no*' by staying strong. This testing procedure is good but not infallible. There is a subjectivity that needs to be honed with experience and training.

The main ingredient for good results is the 'state of awareness' mentioned earlier. This involves both patient and practitioner. The patient who is already 'aware' will learn to respond quickly and reliably. The less aware patient will take a treatment or two to develop that reliability. Fortunately this is not critical. The first few techniques are such that when the practitioner tests for them and there is a problem, the impact on the body is so great that the muscle will simply go weak for a few seconds anyway. Hence, the weakness will still indicate a *yes* answer. The more subtle *yes/no* concept and response is only necessary when we start asking more sophisticated questions in greater depth.

The other part of the 'awareness' equation lies with the BodyTalk practitioner. I stress to my students the absolute importance of developing their 'awareness' so they may 'listen' to the patient objectively. This involves having treatment themselves to train their own system as well as focus on clearing their minds of an agenda. This agenda includes the preconceived ideas and beliefs we may have about treatment and diagnosis; our need to diagnose or label things so we can treat the person 'our' way instead of responding to the patient's own inner wisdom; and prejudging the answer before asking the question, which can lead to shaky responses.

Although it is not a perfect system, muscle testing is the preferred communication technique for BodyTalk because it provides us with immediate feedback and verification, and is simple to use. Its shortcomings are far outweighed by its benefits.

The Art of Muscle Testing

When you are trying out the treatments on the following pages, remember the following guidelines.

The muscle test is relative to the patient. Every patient tests differently. Some people are quite weak to start with because of illness. Remember to test first and then judge the relative degree of weakness. Their *no* answer may feel like a weak muscle, while their *yes* answer can feel even weaker.

Very strong people could have a 20% reduction in strength when you test a trigger point. You may not feel that reduction because even at 80% strength, they still feel strong. For this reason, it is better not to focus on total muscle strength in the test. Try to develop the subtlety to test their 'muscle takeup time.'

A strong, healthy muscle will feel 'solid' when gently tested. Remember to ask the patient to try to hold their current position—not push back. If a muscle is testing 'weak,' it will have a slower 'takeup' time, which means there will be a slight 'sponginess' or 'give' for a small distance before the natural strength of the muscle takes over. This is what we are really looking for. Even the strongest person will have that 'sponginess' or 'shake,' and give you a *yes* answer if you test a muscle while you are contacting malfunctioning trigger points.

My preferred procedure is to test the muscle with the arm at the side. The patient is then asked to keep their arm at their side while the practitioner attempts to pull it away from the body. Remember to keep the patient's arm straight so the shoulder muscles are being used. Then the patient won't be tempted to bend the arm and

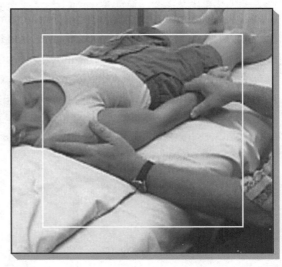

Testing a muscle — the NO answer

35

bring in a second group of muscles.

Now you want to train the inner awareness through the brain into a *yes/no* response. I like to use a little bit of showmanship that helps the patient to focus. I touch their head with one light tap and say, "Resist, give me a no," and pull fairly gently so that the arm is able to stay at the side.

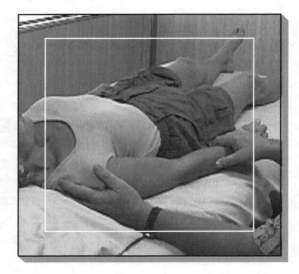

Testing a muscle—the YES answer

I then tap their head lightly twice and say, "Resist, give me a yes," and pull harder so that the arm comes out from the side.

Obviously, this is rigging the results to give the brain feedback so it knows what we want.

After a couple of training runs you will find when you say, "Resist, give me a no," the arm will remain solid with a firm (relative to the patient's strength) pull. Then when you say, "Resist, give me a yes," the patient's arm will go weak even though you are pulling with the same strength as when you asked for a no. This will amaze the patient, and probably you, too, until you get used to the fact that the body is very willing to communicate with you.

Now you have trained the patient and are ready to start communicating with their inner wisdom; asking questions that will always require a *'yes'* or *'no'* answer. This opens up a whole new world of exploration of the bodymind and facilitates the practitioner's ability to ensure that the treatment will take the direction best suited to the occasion.

Linking: Restoring Communication

Linking is the key to the new paradigm of treatment. The practitioner must ask the body what parts need to be linked in order to reestablish good communication and facilitate healing.

The concept of linking is simply the process of:

- Locating a part of the body that has indicated it needs treatment (for example, the liver). It will be found by systematically working through the treatment protocol described in the next chapter. For example, we could arrive at the organ system and ask if organs are a priority. If the answer is yes, each organ is then asked, in turn, if there is a problem. The practitioner is thinking, "Is there a problem?" while they are asking the name of the organ out loud. Heart? *No.* Lung? *No.* Liver? *Yes.*

- Now we want to know to what we link the liver. One usually starts within the same system. So we would ask, "Link to organ?" *Yes.* With the patient's hand on the liver, we would then touch each organ again asking for a link. Heart? *No.* Lung? *No.* Stomach? *No.* Pancreas? *Yes.* We have found a link!

- The patient touches over the liver; the practitioner touches the reflex point for the pancreas with one hand while tapping out the head and sternum. (This is covered in the next section.)

- The patient is retested. Heart to pancreas link a problem? *No.* The link is corrected.

This process goes on with different variations for all the systems. Many times the links will not occur within the system but, instead, to another part of the body. For example, the liver may end up being linked to the adrenal glands or the uterus.

Tapping the Head and Heart

The tapping process is used on the head and sternum (heart) to facilitate the linkage and store it.

This procedure is the most important development in The BodyTalk System™. The technique has been used by some indigenous holistic systems, such as yoga, for centuries. It seemed, however, to have limited application; as it was not understood by Western cultures. It is still not fully understood, but has been shown clinically to have dramatic widespread application in all health systems.

The process of lightly tapping the skull seems to activate the brain centers in a way that causes the brain to consciously reevaluate the state of health in the bodymind. It does this in relation to the linking points that are being isolated. When we just tap the head on its own, nothing significant seems to happen. When we tap the head while we are linking parts of the body (that the innate wisdom has asked to be linked) a great deal happens.

The 'sick' linkage is immediately corrected. (When we retest and ask, "Is there a problem?," the answer is *no*). The rest of the body then readjusts to that correction and a chain of events is set up to bring about balancing and repair to the whole system. This repair is holistic in that the bodymind seems to correct all the factors associated with that illness. For example, if the problem was a low back pain that had an emotional component, i.e. the patient was fearful of some emotional burden, then the emotional component balances and repairs to the tissues of the spinal joints (the patient loses the fear).

It appears when we establish points that need to be linked, and tap the head, we are, essentially, asking the brain to fix the problem. When the heart is tapped, we ask the heart to store and synthesize the correction.

Tapping the Head

The tapping procedure is very light. You barely have to touch the head. It would seem that the impact is not mechanical from the physical tapping. It feels very much like an energy impact—one kinetic energy, the moving fingers, causing an interference node with another energy field, the brain impulses.

The main thing to remember is to make sure that the fingers are spread so that some 'impact' is being made on both hemispheres of the brain. (At least one finger has to touch either side of the head.) At first, the tapping is done for two full breath cycles, alternating between the head and the heart. (See next section.) Once you have treated a number of patients you will begin to 'feel' the changes occurring and the 'shift' of energy happen that indicates a correction. When you feel this, you only need to tap until the correction happens. This could occur in a second or half a minute.

Explaining what the 'shift' feels like is difficult because it is very subjective. I feel it as a tension buildup, much like one feels with an increase in the barometric pressure before a big storm. I can feel this locally around the patient's head and my tapping hand, or sometimes I feel my whole body tense up.

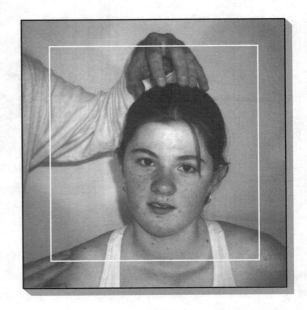

The 'shift' is the release of that tension. The feeling of release after the storm.

It takes a while for a BodyTalk practitioner to develop this sensitivity. Fortunately, it is not necessary for good results. *You simply need to keep tapping for a couple of breaths and the results will occur.*

Tapping the head

Tapping the Sternum (Heart)

The tapping of the sternum appears to correspond to the energic relationship to the heart and heart complex. This technique relates more specifically to the concept of the heart energies. There is significant evidence to show that the heart, in addition to its role of pumping blood, plays a significant role in the distribution of energy in the body. The heart 'pumps' patterns of energy and information to every cell in the body.

It is well known that the electrical potential generated by the heart, identified by an ECG, can be recorded from any site in the body because of volume conduction; a physical mechanism that is not controversial in and of itself.

The heart's conduction of information throughout the system is also clinically verified by the degree of information ascertained from testing the arterial pulses throughout the body.

In BodyTalk and Chinese medicine, the 'pulses' are taken (using different methods) to 'read' information about the state of the body. The pumping of the heart activates energy wave impulses that have the historic dynamic energy memory of all the bodily

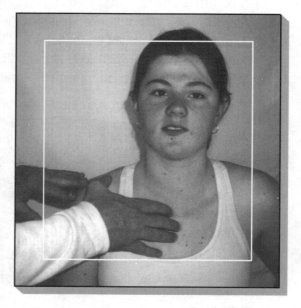

Tapping the sternum

systems superimposed upon them. By placing the fingers on the arterial pulse, the practitioner sets up interference nodes that will contain all this information as long as the practitioner has a system to interpret it. Further, by linking back to the brain or heart (as done in BodyTalk), the memory systems can be altered to correct any anomalies.

In Chinese medicine and bioenergetic psychology, the heart is seen as the central governor and energy organizer of the body. It constantly and dynamically reflects the 'state of affairs' of the body. This is analogous to the concept of collective, dynamic, interactive, historic memory or consciousness. It further transpires that if one can change the memory, the health and dynamic consciousness of the entire bodymind system can be modified

The term 'knowing things by heart' shows society's innate understanding of the dynamics of the bodymind. All cells store information. The heart is intimately and dynamically connected to all the cells and organs because of the centrality of its location and connections.

Consider the ramifications of heart transplants in light of this information. One could assume from the above discussion that the heart recipient would receive some of the historical aspects the donor has processed and stored. The body of the recipient has just lost its own central dynamical energy processor and memory. This has been replaced by foreign patterns that will not correspond to the established patterns innate to the recipient's body. Whether they are sick (the need for a transplant) or reasonably healthy, they are still the established memory patterns of that individual ego. Surely, much of the rejection process, manifested as chemical and immune reactions, would make more sense if they were seen as interactive memory battles producing the manifestation of chemical rejection.

There is an increasing amount of evidence that points to the validity of this transferred memory concept. Consider the case of Claire Sylvia:

In her book, A Change of Heart, *Sylvia, a former dancer, describes how her life went through a variety of changes after receiving a heart-lung transplant. For example, six weeks after the operation, she was allowed to drive again, and she drove straight to Kentucky Fried Chicken, a place she had never been before. Then this fit, thin, dancer ordered fried chicken nuggets! Later, she learned that the 18-year-old whose heart and lungs were now living inside her had had a fondness for chicken nuggets. At the time of the man's death, uneaten chicken nuggets had been found stuffed inside the pocket of his leather jacket.*

By tapping the heart we seem to be helping the bodymind superimpose 'what should be' in place of 'what has been' going on, thereby ensuring that the procedure will last. It appears the tapping inputs dynamic kinetic energy into the static memory contained in the heart complex (which includes the heart chakra), and causes the bodymind to reestablish a new memory under the newly corrected system. Remember, we have just corrected the system by tapping the head while we held the linking points.

Again the tapping is light and can be done over the sternum. Lately I have found that it is preferable to tap more to the left of the sternum over the heart. This is not always possible in some cultures because of possible contact with the breast.

IN SUMMARY:
- Tapping the head repairs the linkage.
- Tapping the heart stores the changes to make them permanent.

Exaggerated Breathing

Exaggerated breathing is often used to help the body locate and target the corrections.

Hatha yoga says that if a person has perfect breath, they will have perfect health. The BodyTalk System™ agrees with this statement and utilizes the immense importance of the full breath cycle in treatments and, more importantly, to ensure the treatment lasts.

The breath cycle can be divided into many functions. Most of these are well known in human physiology and will not be covered here. I am more interested in discussing some of the little known, but vitally important, functions of the breath cycle.

The breath cycle is one of our main energy pumps.

Energy accumulates in the lungs from the air we breathe and the food energy sent up to the lungs from the digestive system (a principle of Chinese medicine). This energy is then pumped through the meridian system via the lung meridian that starts in the lungs. The more powerful our breath cycle, the more powerful the flow of energy through the meridians.

The whole body rocks with our breath cycle.

As we breathe in and out, our whole body moves in synchronicity with that movement. The muscles expand and contract to pump the blood returning to the heart and pump the lymph (our sewerage system) around the body.

Our cranial bones make very small movements that change the pressure inside the cranial vault and cause the cerebrospinal fluid to circulate. This keeps the nervous system bathed in the fluids vital to its function.

Each vertebrae in the spine rocks in synchronicity with the breathing cycle, maintaining healthy functioning and the integrity of the spine and spinal cord.

The skin breathes air in and out as our lungs breathe. A large amount of the air we take into our body is through the skin, not the lungs!

The breath cycle influences the heartbeat.

The yogis have long demonstrated that by controlling their breath, they can control the beating of their heart. This is very important in BodyTalk because we utilize this relationship to bring about lasting changes in the treatment. We do this by imprinting the changes we make onto the heart energy system.

The brain uses the breath cycle to scan the body.

This is another yoga principle that has immense relevance to BodyTalk. Each time we breathe in and out, the brain scans all of the frequencies of the body. As we breathe out, the scanning goes down the frequencies from highest to lowest. As we breathe in, the reverse happens.

From science we know that our body is, ultimately, just a bundle of energy made up of different frequencies. The slower the frequencies, the denser the parts. Bones, for example, represent the slower frequencies of the body; blood is a higher frequency; meridian energy is higher still. The emotions and thoughts represent some of the highest frequencies found in the bodymind complex.

Each of these frequencies are contained within systems of energy that 'hold' the bodymind together. There are systems within systems within systems. Each of these has dynamic relationships with all the other systems within the bodymind and outside of it as well. Whenever any of these systems fail, disharmony occurs. This becomes evident in the specific frequencies associated with that system.

During each breath cycle, the brain scans these systems to establish if any are malfunctioning. *How well it can do this, depends upon how healthy our breathing cycle is.*

If our breathing cycle is restricted, our brain and heart energy will not be able to correctly ascertain the state of our health and will make mistakes. *If the brain doesn't know what is wrong — it can't fix it!*

Examples

Breathing out—the act of 'letting go'.

Low frequency diseases are usually chronic bone or muscle diseases such as arthritis, or chronic muscular degenerative diseases. In clinical observations, patients in chronic pain with arthritis rarely ever fully breathe out. If they try to, they suddenly experience pain. They breathe shallowly to stop themselves from getting in touch with that discomfort.

Psychologically, arthritis sufferers tend to be people who spent their lives driving themselves and/or remaining fixed in rigid belief systems about life and how it should be lived. A rigid mind leads to a rigid body. 'Driven' people will rarely allow themselves to fully let go. The act of breathing all the way out is a characteristic of being able to fully let go to life. If you spend your life living in stress, the body stops breathing out fully and the brain stops scanning those lower frequencies. This means that if we are developing arthritis, for whatever reason, the brain will not fully recognize the problem. Instead, it will allow the degenerative process to continue without significant intervention.

Breathing in—getting in touch with life.

When we breathe in, we are entering the higher frequencies of thought and emotion. People who don't breathe in fully do not allow full interaction with their emotional and mental processes. An emotionally disturbed person will not breathe all the way in because they inwardly know that it will cause them to suddenly get in touch with deep feelings. This will eventually lead to the brain not recognizing the emotional or mental state; resulting in disease processes establishing themselves without intervention and correction by the brain's healing processes.

When we treat someone with BodyTalk, we often ask the patient to take a deep breath in and out, to ensure that the brain is getting fully in touch with the problem we are highlighting with our techniques.

44

Getting Permission

Veils of Resistance

In BodyTalk we are consulting the innate wisdom for guidance on how to treat the patient. The actual treatment, however, is conducted by the various parts of the body and the states of consciousness that control them.

The bodymind complex is simply a range of frequencies clustered together into various 'groups' of consciousness. At this stage we are concerned with the three major frequency groups that make up the bodymind:

THE BODY
the lower range of frequencies

THE MIND
the midrange of frequencies

THE SOUL
the upper range of frequencies relating to all spiritual aspects

The mind is best divided into the:

CONSCIOUS MIND
all those things of which we can think

UNCONSCIOUS MIND
those things beyond conscious thought processes

This now gives us four divisions of the body:

BODY
CONCIOUS MIND
UNCONCIOUS MIND
SOUL

Each of these divisions can be regarded as a state of consciousness effectively controlled by it own separate 'Ego' state. Each of these 'Ego' states have a relationship to the whole bodymind complex but still have 'local' authority.

There is often an assumption by practitioners that once a person has agreed to treatment means they have given permission to be treated. Our experience in BodyTalk is that this is often the case on certain levels only. For example, the patient's mind and soul may be ready to be treated but not the body. If this is so, then the patient will respond poorly on the physical level which will slow down or, in some cases, stop the long term results.

This is true in all healing systems and can account for poor results even when the system seems to be working at the time of treatment. For example, if the surgeon has not specifically obtained permission from the body 'Ego' of a patient, the body will often react unfavorably to the surgery and have complications that were unexpected. In another case, an emotional treatment on someone whose unconscious mind has not given permission will stop the treatment from lasting or cause adverse reactions and complications.

In a nutshell, *you need to ask the body for permission to treat it at each of the four levels of 'Ego' awareness before you proceed with a BodyTalk treatment*, or any other health care modality. I have found that when this is done, the results improve dramatically.

CASE HISTORY:

Jan had been having BodyTalk treatments for several problems including stress, ovarian cysts, and emotional problems relating to her husband.

Her original response to the BodyTalk treatment was very good. She was more relaxed, emotionally stable, getting on better with her husband and sleeping better with more energy when she woke up. However, her ovarian cysts had not responded to treatment and she was still having severe pain with ovulation and the ovaries were very tender to the touch. During the sessions I could get very few linkages to the ovaries. They seemed to be a very low priority.

When the importance of the permission concept became apparent to me, I asked each 'Ego' for permission to treat. I was given permission to treat from the mind, unconscious mind, and the soul. I was denied permission from the body. Although she was happily my patient, her body 'Ego' did not want to be treated! I then used the technique to correct this and obtained permission.

The BodyTalk treatment that followed gave me vastly different link-ages to the ovaries and the response was dramatic. Jan felt constant activity in and around her ovaries for days and her cysts cleared up completely.

I have found that even the cooperative 'Ego' parts prefer to be formally asked permission to treat. This sets the stage for the respect of the patient's body and, therefore, its cooperation in working with the guidance of the innate wisdom. It should be noted here that the innate wisdom does not have to be asked permission because it is beyond 'Ego' expression and will always be working for the highest good of the patient. The other aspects of the individual are polarized energy patterns. They are consciousness centers subject to the distortions of the conscious and unconscious minds.

Asking Permission

Once you have established your *Yes/No* protocol at the start of the treatment, you then ask:

"Do I have permission to treat your body?"

"Do I have permission to treat your conscious mind?

"Do I have permission to treat your unconscious mind?"

"Do I have permission to treat your soul?"

If the answer is *yes* to all questions then you have full permission and cooperation from the body.

If the answer is *no* to any one or more of them, then there is a veil of resistance to your treatment. This means, for some reason, that particular aspect of the bodymind is out of sync and needs to be synchronized with the rest of the bodymind.

Treatment

Have the patient physically write down permission to treat the particular part that responded with a *no* answer on a piece of paper. (For example: *I Jan give permission for John to treat my body.*)

47

Place the piece of paper in the patient's navel and ask if you can treat this statement. If the answer is *yes*, then tap out the head and sternum while the patient takes two deep breaths and thinks about the statement.

Now ask the initial question again:

"Do I have permission to treat your body?" (Or whichever it was.)

If the answer is *yes*, move on.

If the answer is *no*—and that will be rare—then I suggest you don't treat the patient and send them to a BodyTalk practitioner who will know what to do. When this happens to a BodyTalk practitioner they use the environmental treatment to harmonize the patient with the practitioner. In these cases either the patient or the practitioner is not feeling at ease at some level, with the other. This needs to be resolved at this stage or the patient/practitioner relationship will be unsettled and limited.

If there was originally a second *no* response, then repeat the treatment procedure for next 'Ego.'

Once permission is granted at all four levels you then ask one more question:

"Are any other permissions needed?"

If the answer is *yes* then you will ask:

"Do you need to give yourself permission to get better?"

The *yes* answer will show the patient that, at the deepest level, there was an aspect of them that really wasn't ready to get better. This needs to be tapped out.

Have the patient say, *"I give myself permission to get better,"* while you tap out the head and sternum.

Retest to ensure that it has worked.

Once this is done you are free to confidently proceed with your treatment with the knowledge that you will have full cooperation from the patient at the four main levels of 'Ego' awareness.

CHAPTER

8

What Disorders Can BodyTalk Help?

AN OVERVIEW

THIS BOOK IS NOT DESIGNED TO COVER EVERYTHING IN THE BODYTALK System™. In this chapter I will present the general treatment protocol outline that BodyTalk practitioners use as a guideline in practice. In the next chapter I will make comments on each section and give some related case examples. The protocol is divided into Module 1 and Module 2. This indicates the subject matter covered in the two Modules taught in BodyTalk workshops. They can be taken as separate weekends (an evening and two days) or an intensive week long workshop that combines both Modules.

Later in the book I will be covering many of the techniques that are safe, simple, and very effective for many common health problems. You can try out The BodyTalk System™ and see for yourself why BodyTalk is truly a health care system for the 21st century.

In the first outline, the sections that are italicized are the sections that will be covered in detail later in the book.

Module 1

I. **EGT (Essential general treatments)**

    A. *SB joint*

    B. Switching

    C. *Basic cortex correction*

    D. *Hydration*

    E. *Scars and clothing*

    F. Basic brain balancing

II. **Organs**

    A. *Linking the organs (lungs, heart, liver, gall bladder, stomach, pancreas, small intestine, colon, kidney, bladder)*

    B. Linking to the central nervous system

III. **Endocrine**

    A. Linking the endocrine glands (pineal, pituitary/hypo thalamus, thyroid, thymus, spleen, adrenals, ovaries, testes)

    B. Linking to the central nervous system

IV. **Body parts**

    A. Linking all the body parts

V. Body Chemistry (saliva)

A. *Treating viruses, infections, parasites, food intolerances, accumulated toxins, and allergies*

B. Linking them to the rest of the system and emotions where necessary

VI. Emotional

A. Present
   1. Heart (self-esteem, love issues)
   2. Pelvis (sensuality and sexuality issues)
   3. Body image, body acceptance
   4. Relationships
   5. Current life situations

B. Past
   1. Lifetime periods (specific years in the life)
   2. Past relationships (mother, father, family, others)
   3. Childbirth, fetal life
   4. Specific incidents and events
   5. Specific fears and phobias

C. Specific
   1. Treating the emotion behind one of the specific physical imbalances or body parts
   2. Treating the emotion behind specific injuries
   3. Treating the emotion behind specific diseases

Module 2

VII. **Cellular repair**

   A. Vaccines (damage caused by vaccines)

   B. Hereditary genetics (treatment of aspects of hereditary genetic diseases where possible)

   C. Accumulated cellular destruction (repairing the damage caused during the lifetime by various chemical, physical, or emotional traumas)

VII. **Extrinsic balancing: The Reciprocals**

   A. Upper Body - Lower Body

     1. upper shoulder/iliac crest

     2. shoulder tip/hip

     3. shoulder front/front of hip

     4. shoulder back/ back of hip

     5. elbow/knee

     6. wrist/ankle

     7. navel/coccyx

   B. Head - Body

     1. vomer/xiphoid

     2. temporal bone/innominate bone

     3. zygoma/pubic crest

     4. mouth/navel

     5. ear/axilla

     6. eye/breast

C. Head - Spinal Complex
  1. TMJ/sacroiliac joint
  2. sphenoid/coccyx
  3. occiput/sacrum
  4. styloid/lumbosacral
  5. upper spine/lower spine

IX. Lymphatic

A. Linking the zygoma to the lymph glands of the neck, sub-clavicular area, breast, splenic sub-diaphragm area, abdomen, groin

X. The Nervous and Circulatory Systems

A. Linking the brain to body parts, organs, and endocrines for nerve flow to, or within, the part
B. Linking the heart (circulation) to body parts, organs, and endocrines for blood flow to, or within, the part

XI. Energy Systems

A. *Linking the seven chakras*
B. *Vivaxis*
C. Meridians and sugar balance
  1. balance the 12 meridian pulses
  2. balance the sugar pulses
  3. the pancreas reflex point

XII. Musculo-skeletal

A. Intrinsic treatment of the fascia for each of the body parts indicated
B. Treatment of specific sports injuries and arthritic joints

XIII. Environmental

Checking for links between the patient and factors in his/her environment; environmental factors include people, animals, chemicals, physical objects, and stressful situations

1. Linking the physical body to the environment
2. Linking the emotions to the environment

CHAPTER

9

What Disorders Can BodyTalk Help?

MODULE ONE

IN THIS CHAPTER I WILL EXAMINE THE TREATMENT PROTOCOL AGAIN BUT in more depth and with examples and case histories.

EGT (Essential General Treatments)

These are considered the Essential General Treatments that begin every BodyTalk treatment. As you will see when I discuss them, they prepare the patient for any form of treatment by correcting the essential elements necessary for the body to heal. I firmly believe they are essential for all therapies. If any health care practitioner of any modality prepared their patient using these techniques, I am certain their results would be dramatically improved since they would then have a bodymind ready for therapy.

I have received reports from practitioners that constantly affirm this statement. Chiropractic adjustments hold better and correct easier; acupuncture treatments work faster; homeopathic remedies act quicker; drugs respond better with fewer side effects; patients recover from surgery quicker and with less complications; massage and rolfing have far greater impact; rehabilitation is faster; emotions, phobias, and mental disorders respond to therapy faster and less traumatically. Why this occurs will become obvious as you read on.

SB Joint

This important technique will be covered in more detail later in this book. Briefly, this technique improves the breathing pattern of the body by releasing the critical sections of the skull that move in synchronicity with the breathing cycle. When measured with a respirometer, it often shows a 30% or greater respiratory output after treatment. It also affects the function of the pituitary gland and, therefore, the whole endocrine system.

CASE HISTORY:

Jenny was attending a BodyTalk workshop and routinely did the SB joint correction in class. She immediately became excited and loudly proclaimed "I can breathe". She then explained that as long as she could remember, breathing in deeply required a lot of effort. She was not really asthmatic but was often short of breath and found deep breathing a chore. As soon as the SB joint correction was done, deep breathing was effortless and, to Jenny, exhilarating!

CASE HISTORY:

Susan was 12 years old and had the body of an 8 year old. At eight years her pituitary stopped functioning. Although she was on a cocktail of hormones prescribed by an endocrinologist, she was still gravely ill and weak. After the SB correction she felt shooting pains inside her head in the approximate location of the pituitary gland. Within two months her pituitary gland was functioning normally and her body was on the process of total recovery.

Switching

Our left brain is the part of the brain found in both cortices that is considered to handle the normal linear functions of the brain, routine calculations, and day to day simple conscious activity. The right brain involves intuition, creativity, daydreaming, visualization, and complex brain activity.

Normally, the body is constantly switching back and forth between the two 'brains' and we go smoothly from simple functions to complex reasoning and visualization. When we overdo it and over stress ourselves, the body 'switches' and stops that smooth transition and we seem to 'lose it.' Our thoughts become cloudy and our focus poor. This is the brain's way of telling us that we need a break; need to replenish our glucose levels and rest.

For some people, the stress threshold that causes switching is too close to normal activity. These people 'switch' too easily and find themselves constantly losing focus and concentration. Even the stress of having to take an exam will cause them to 'switch' and perform badly. This is common with students or people who work in stressful, performance related jobs.

This technique improves the threshold that causes the switching. Once it is corrected, the brain switches less easily and the patient's performance capacity is increased. This technique is vital in health care because the patient is often stressed from the disease, or even the stress of going to a practitioner. When the body is in the 'switched' mode, it has poor focus and healing ability. The patient will therefore not respond appropriately to the treatment given, often confusing the treatments and giving unusual results or reactions. By 'unswitching' the patient at the beginning of a treatment session, the practitioner can be sure that the body will respond appropriately to the techniques administered or prescribed.

Basic Cortex Correction

This is one of the fundamental techniques and is used, in various ways, in BodyTalk. Essentially, it is about repairing the brain from the perspective of communication between the two hemispheres.

By balancing and correcting any faults between the two hemispheres the innate wisdom of the body requests, we are able to help the body recover from many serious diseases and malfunctions. We also greatly enhance the general functioning of the brain and the circulation of blood, cerebrospinal fluid, and nerves within it. One of the most common expressions I hear, after correction, is that the patient suddenly "feels clearer in the head," or "has a greater sense of wellbeing."

Once this is corrected, the brain will be far more responsive to any therapy. I personally would never touch a patient until I have at least corrected the basic cortices. I have found it to be extremely significant. This technique will be covered—enthuasiastically—in more detail later.

Hydration

Water therapy is often talked about but little understood. We give lip service to the importance of water intake, yet most people think that simply means 'fluid intake'. They base this on the supposition that all fluid contains water and therefore helps to supply the water needs of the body. The fact is that coffee, tea, some herbal teas, and sodas contain caffeine or caffeine-like substances. Caffeine is a dehydrating agent that increases the function of the kidneys causing dehydration. Therefore, the drinking of these beverages without supplementary pure water has the ultimate effect of dehydrating the tissues and cells.

Many people seem to think of water as merely a solvent, a packaging material, and means for transportation of other substances in the body. They place more emphasis on proteins, minerals and vitamins. The fact is water is vital in energy production in the cells, metabolism, emotional synthesis, lymph circulation, and neurotransmission.

Many patients will tell you they drink plenty of water because they realize its importance. Some of these patients seem to have fluid retention because they have far too much fluid in their body. Yet, when I test them for hydration, the test says they are very dehydrated! The other problem is that drinking large glasses of water often doesn't rehydrate them—it just makes them feel sick. This is typical of the reaction of the person found in the desert who is given a large amount of water: the body reacts badly.

This hydration problem occurs because of poor osmosis in the cell membranes. Much of the fluid is staying between the cells and not transporting through the cell membrane into the intracellular space where the action occurs. The water is in the body, but it is not being used in the right places.

This simple hydration technique corrects that problem and helps the body to utilize the water effectively. It is, therefore, fundamental to any treatment system since the body cannot possibly respond effectively to any treatment when the body is dehydrated. The technique is taught later in this book.

CASE HISTORY:

Gary had chronic headaches, a pressure feeling in his head, and tiredness. He noted that he always seemed thirsty and that whenever he drank alcohol or sodas, his headaches increased in intensity. He had read about the water factor and had greatly increased his water intake. This improved his condition greatly but it never lasted. He constantly needed huge amounts of water to relieve his condition. He was putting on weight with fluid retention!

After a BodyTalk hydration treatment, his body return to normal, his thirst, headaches, and tiredness went away. All he needed was a normal intake of water.

Scars and Clothing

This techniques treats unhealthy scars and identifies whether or not certain articles of clothing or jewelry are detrimental to the health of the patient; or if they could be interfering with the effectiveness of the treatment.

Unhealthy scars block the flow of energy along the meridian energy pathways and inhibit the function of all the areas supplied by that meridian. Unhealthy scars will also upset the energic hologram of the body by interfering with the general balance of energy throughout the body.

Many health problems have started when a scar has partially blocked the flow of energy through the body. Scars usually do not heal well when there is an emotional upset going on at the time the cut is formed, whether it be from an accident or surgery. This is one of the most overlooked and least understood aspects of health care. I have personally treated thousands of scars with amazing results. Often the scar treatment would be all that is necessary to correct the health problem. This simple, yet very important, treatment will be covered later and I feel sure it will be one of your favorites!

CASE HISTORY:

Jim cut his finger when he offered to help his wife in the kitchen. It was only a nick at the base of his finger nail on the first finger. It infuriated him because it would not stop bleeding and it ruined the potatoes he had peeled. He stormed out of the kitchen and the bleeding eventually stopped.

About a month later Jim started having problems with his intestines with pain and tenderness. This eventually worsened and he saw his doctor. After another few months the diagnosis of irritable bowel syndrome was made and he was on constant medication. After three years he was told he may need a section of his bowel removed as the only means of giving him relief.

During a consequent treatment his body told me, through the muscle testing feedback, about the scar. I would never have seen it because it was too small. I noticed that the scar was directly over the acupuncture point CO1. This is the first point on the colon meridian in acupuncture and can greatly influence the bowel. The scar was treated and the body was satisfied that the problem would be fixed. Within a month most of Jim's pain and irritation had gone. Within three months he was symptom free and has stayed that way.

Basic Brain Balancing

The basic brain techniques involve balancing and linking the brain in three major sections: the cortices, the limbic brain, and the reptilian brain. This is very important for coordinating the general functions of the brain and its ability to control the bodymind complex. In advanced BodyTalk we go into the balancing of the brain and repair of brain function in depth. This part of BodyTalk treatment is rapidly becoming a major part of advanced BodyTalk practice.

CASE HISTORY:

Gary was 12 years old and had a great deal of difficulty with coordination. He was very limited in sports and writing skills. He even found it an effort to open and close his hands quickly. I was directed to his brain by his innate wisdom and found that the motor section of the brain on the left side did not seem to be linking well with the cerebellum. After the link was tapped out, Gary had improved speed in opening and closing his hands within five minutes. Over the next few weeks, all motor coordination functions improved significantly.

CASE HISTORY:

Jenny was a 50 year old mother of seven children who came to me for back problems. During her routine treatment I was directed to link two sections of her brain—the left sensory section to the right frontal lobe of the brain. After a few minutes Jenny became excited and proclaimed that her brain was functioning again.

She explained that ever since the birth of her second child her brain has felt like it was in a fog. She could not think clearly and secretly feared the onset of Alzheimer's disease. She never told me about it because, after so many years, she had accepted it as a 'normal' condition for her. Despite this attitude, her innate wisdom had directed me to correct the problem and give her a new lease on life.

Organs

- Specific treatment of the liver, gall bladder, stomach, heart, small intestine, colon, and bladder;
- *Linking the organs—lungs, heart, liver, gall bladder, stomach, pancreas, small intestine, colon, kidney, bladder;*
- Linking to the central nervous system

At this stage of treatment we enter the main 'physical medicine' phase. In this section the BodyTalk practitioner is balancing the relationship and synchronicity between the organs. They are also linked to the central nervous system to ensure a good nerve supply and to the heart to ensure good circulation both to the organ and within it. The basics of this section are covered in this book.

CASE HISTORY:

Ann had just been through two weeks of a bad virus and infection of the lung and upper respiratory tract. (She did not have BodyTalk for it!) Now she was complaining to a neighbor that she simply could not shake off the last of the illness. She had a cough and congestion in the lungs, constipation, tiredness, and headaches. The neighbor had attended the Module 1 BodyTalk workshop. She proceeded to give Ann a BodyTalk treatment that, among other things, balanced her lung to her colon and spleen. Her adrenals were also balanced to her liver. The recovery was dramatic. By the next day Ann was healthy.

CASE HISTORY:

Ken had chronic digestive problems, especially in digesting fats. He was always bloated and felt heavy and 'stuck' in the intestines. The BodyTalk System™ established there was poor communication between is gall bladder and small intestine. After this was tapped out, the secretions from his gall bladder normalized and all symptoms disappeared.

Endocrine

- *Linking the endocrine glands (pineal, pituitary/hypothalamus thyroid, thymus, spleen, adrenals, ovaries, testes)*
- Linking to the central nervous system

The endocrines are treated in the same way as organs. Once again we see the biggest problem with endocrines is that they are not synchronized in their activities. This synchronicity is more vital in the endocrine system than any other system. The balance of secretions between the pituitary, ovaries, and adrenals is vital for such things as regulation of the menstrual cycle, stress handling, mood changes, depression, food cravings, and dozens of other factors.

CASE HISTORY:

Jane had a chronic problem with handling stress. Everything got to her and somedays she felt like she would 'explode' if the phone rang just once more. Everything was much worse between ovulation and her menstrual flow. The stress kept her awake at night, screaming at the kids, unresponsive to her husband sexually, and her stomach felt knotted.

During her BodyTalk treatment, her innate wisdom asked the pituitary to be linked to the adrenals and then the adrenals to the ovaries. Finally her liver was linked to her heart. The relief started on the treatment table. After two more treatments she was symptom free and has remained that way for five months at time of writing.

Body Parts

- Linking the sense organs (eyes, ears, nose, mouth), hair, teeth, throat, breasts, diaphragm, skin, internal connective tissue, uterus, prostate, genitals, buttocks, and nails;
- Specific local treatment of the eyes, breast and diaphragm

In this section links are found to all the other systems and body parts beyond the organs and endocrines. These connections give the innate wisdom access to a much greater variety of links for balancing the body. This is a fascinating section of BodyTalk since we see links that are not always explainable from current traditional knowledge.

In my own research, I try to understand the nature of the link in relation to the symptoms of the patient. Many times I can explain them with conventional physiology, on other occasions I need Chinese medical philosophy to find an explanation. In other cases, bioenergetic psychology provides the answer. In some cases, I am still looking for explanations.

One of the more fascinating linking system involves cases where a body part such as the knee is linked to an organ or endocrine. For example, the patient may have a link between the kidneys and the knee. Further analysis shows that the patient has a history of reoccurring kidney problems linked to emotional stresses particularly relating to fear of life and the patient's ability to cope with their current life situation.

By combining a knowledge of Chinese philosophy and bioenergetic psychology, the explanation of this and other links to different organs becomes obvious. As an example, I will give you an explanation of the workings and relationships of four of the main joints of the body from this perspective.

I AM THE ELBOW

You may think that I am only here to enable you to bend your arm. I do much more than that. My state of health is a reflection of the state of health physically and mentally of many areas of the body. I can, therefore, tell you a great deal about yourself.

Six meridians (acupuncture energy channels) flow through me. The meridians of the lung, pericardium, and heart flow along my inner aspect. The outer aspect is controlled by the meridians of the colon, triple heater, and small intestine. When certain attributes of these meridians are dysfunctional because of things you do, it will reflect in my well-being.

The inside meridians are Yin meridians and the dysfunctional aspects which relate to me are negative reactive tendencies, poor adaptability (lung), inability to protect and nurture the heart emotionally (pericardium), restricted awareness of life, sadness or depression (heart). When any of these aspects are unbalanced, I will often give you a sign (symptom) along the inside of my arm.

The most common symptom is pain or tenderness. In conventional medical diagnosis, pain along the inside of the arm sometimes indicates heart problems. The studies of bioenergetics and Chinese medicine say this can specifically point to heart problems developing from lack of awareness, chronic sadness or depression. Lack of awareness is reflected in a lifestyle that is detrimental to the heart. Chronic stress, poor dietary habits and repressed emotional turmoil

63

can take their toll on the physical and emotional heart. Sometimes, the lack of awareness relates to a lack or neglect of spiritual awareness. People going through major spiritual changes which they don't understand or aren't synthesizing properly, will often suffer pain, tenderness or swelling on the inside aspect of the elbow. This is particularly common in the case of 'spiritual emergency'; where the person has been inwardly fighting their destiny and refusing to accept the changes that are happening in their life that could be putting them back on track.

The outside meridians are Yang meridians and relate to the psychological concepts of being intellectually over-challenged, inability to differentiate good/bad, right/wrong (small intestine), letting go and forgiveness (colon).

The small intestine separates the good, nutritious elements of our food and absorbs them into the blood stream. The waste products then move on to the colon. Psychologically, the small intestine relates to our intellect and, in particular, to our ability to differentiate good and bad, and right and wrong in life. (The intellectual process could be defined as a processing of information with discernment between what is useful and what isn't.) A malfunctioning small intestine can impair our intellectual ability to judge life in a positive way. We tend to develop negative belief systems and attitudes and our clarity of thought is muddied. Conversely, long-term poor judgment and negative thinking will impair the function of the small intestine and its ability to extract the good nutrients and pass on the waste. When this occurs, even a good diet will be poorly metabolized. Symptomatically, this will reflect in pain and tenderness on the outside aspect of the elbow.

The waste food products from the small intestine pass down to the colon for elimination. The colon is one of the main organs responsible for eliminating waste from our body. Psychologically, our ability or inability to eliminate waste from our body reflects our ability to eliminate the waste parts of our life. Our inability to forgive others and ourselves for things that have happened in our lives, gives rise to functional disturbances of the colon. People who refuse to forgive themselves, or others, because of some negative (wasted) event, will end up with chronic bowel problems. Similarly, our ability to "let go to the process of life" is also reflected in the health of our bowel. We see people who are unable to "go with the flow" ending up with chronic constipation or problems relating to irritable bowel syndrome. Conversely, people going through a life crisis who feel they are losing control of their lives, often find the "bottom falls out of their life" and they develop diarrhea.

Not "flowing with life" and struggling against that flow is one of the most common causes of chronic elbow problems. The so-called "tennis elbow," which does not quickly respond to treatment, is often related to a chronic bowel problem. Very often, effective treatment involves physically treating the colon or counseling the patient on the concepts of letting go and forgiveness. Local symptomatic treatment of the elbow will prove ineffective in the long term unless the underlying causes are treated.

When the "tennis elbow" is also associated with chronic constipation, dramatic relief can often be forthcoming with colonic irrigation. Observation often shows the etiology of a "tennis elbow" being that of repetitive movement. This also fits into the picture. Constant repetitive movement will eventually be interpreted by the mind as a chronic tendency to be inflexible in life or "in a rut." Hence, the body will eventually send us a symptom to say that we are loosing our spontaneity in the form of elbow inflexibility.

Chiropractors have often had good results treating "tennis elbow" by mobilizing the spine and muscles in the neck. Biomechanically this will free the nerve supply to the elbow. Energically it will encourage energy flow down the arm. Psychologically the neck, if tense, reflects rigidity in attitude. By mobilizing this rigidity, the patient is more able to let go generally. This, in turn, will promote the eventual correction of the elbow symptom.

The key word for the elbow is flexibility. Our elbows reflect our flexibility to life; an ability to adapt and be spontaneous without getting bogged down and constipated by life. The more flexible we are, the more we are able to flow with life, forgive, differentiate right and wrong, intellectually process life, and adapt to our surroundings. If our elbows are losing their flexibility through pain, swelling, arthritis or injury, then we are being told to look at those aspects of our life relating to flexibility.

I AM THE KNEE

I allow you the flexibility to bend down and move around. I am controlled primarily by your kidney energies. The kidney energies relate to fear and willpower.

I have always been a strong metaphor for you in your life. I represent your willpower. When, as a child, you wanted to summon your willpower in defiance, you would lock your knees. You learned the metaphor of bending your knees in submission to your God, your leader or your victor. When you have issues around your willpower, they will reflect in disturbances in my function.

You use willpower to help overcome fear—the other energy of the kidneys. These two opposing forces within the kidneys represent the two opposing forces of the fire and water balance in the dualistic yang/yin functions of the kidneys.

When you experience extreme fear, your knees will go weak. Fortunately, that doesn't happen too often in modern society. Something else happens though, that can be more destructive because of its insidious nature. In modern society, the biggest fear is the fear of coping. Fear of coping with money, work, relationships, health, etc. When you live with this kind of fear, I will be weakened and prone to injury. If it is prolonged over a long time and is coupled with weakened willpower to overcome the fear, then my brain will strengthen me by making me inflexible and rigid. You will call this arthritis.

The inner side of me is controlled by the spleen/pancreas. So if you hurt my medial ligaments, then you are worrying about something you are not coping with. (The spleen/pancreas controls worry.)

My outer side is controlled by the gall bladder so if you injure that part, you are fearful of making a decision about something.

The cruciate ligament deep inside my center relates to the deepest aspect of willpower — the will to survive. When I am injured, you are usually deeply questioning aspects of your very life and existence. This does not mean you are suicidal, just that you are deeply questioning your life, its direction, and your will to follow through and do what needs to be done in your life.

The bladder controls the back of me. The bladder meridian profoundly influences the central nervous system and activity. When that part of me is injured, it usually relates to your allowing your willpower to become over controlled by your nervous system. You become rigid, inflexible and fearful underneath. You 'stand up' for yourself in too reactive a way.

If your hamstrings are also involved, the colon (letting go) controls them. That means that your are fearful of letting go of the 'stance' you are taking—to your detriment. Usually, I start aching in the back when you are going through a period of your life when your beliefs are being challenged and you are afraid to let go of them.

When we treat these joints with BodyTalk we are treating all the aspects of the joints—physical and psychological. By doing this, The BodyTalk System™ is providing a truly holistic approach to the treatment of disease. The BodyTalk System™ takes a dynamical systems approach in regulating all aspects of the dynamic interactions of the various bodymind systems. By establishing better communication, the system is able to correctly ascertain all the ingredients necessary to regain balance and harmony in function.

Once again, the BodyTalk treatment for correcting these important functions is simple.

I AM THE WRIST

I am a complex character because I have such close ties to the hand, which is the most complex and expressive part of the body. I have to be very flexible and mobile so I have eight small bones to give me that incredible flexibility and precision of movement.

I actually need a lot of intelligence to do that, so it is little wonder that the stomach primarily controls me. The stomach represents the conscious mind. (You think with your stomach.) When you start thinking too much and especially when your thinking becomes rigid and narrow-minded, then I become rigid. When your mind is unwilling to reach out to the world with open flexibility, then I will tighten up and restrict the movement in your hands. Your hands will start to withdraw and contract. You will call this 'carpal tunnel.'

If you can't 'stomach' your life and what is happening around you, then you will start having indigestion and I will ache and degenerate. If you have powerful ideas that aren't being expressed, then I will store them in ganglions. When you overwork your brain and strain your eyes (an aspect of which is also controlled by the stomach) such as you do on a computer, I will get sore. You will call it 'repetitive strain injury.' This is funny since there are many other activities that will strain your wrist, but the injury doesn't happen because you aren't working your conscious mind, which is what really agitates me.

The colon and lungs control that part of me near the base of the thumb. The lungs relate to stored or over-reactive grief. The colon is the organ of letting go (see 'I Am The Elbow'). So when I hurt there, it usually means there is some kind of grief in your life that you are not letting go of.

The outside of me, near the little finger, is controlled by the small intestine. The small intestine is smarter than the stomach (conscious mind). It relates directly to our intellect at the highest level. Recent discoveries in neurophysiology show that there are large amounts of brain peptides in the linings of the small intestine. (But then I don't need science to tell me that.)

The small intestine processes food by extracting the good and letting the bad pass on to the colon. The intellect processes thoughts into good (useful) and bad (useless). It discerns and discards. Interestingly, the main brain peptides found in the small intestine are related to the limbic system of the brain where emotions are processed. Very few intellectual decisions about right and wrong are made without emotional interference.

The small intestine also absorbs strong emotions that the body is trying to eliminate. This can be felt and heard as the gurgling in your tummy when you are upset.

When you are not processing the right and wrong in your life correctly and not allowing your emotions to be absorbed and eliminated through the small intestine, then I will start giving you pain and will be easily injured. Your hands will often go numb, ache and have poor circulation, because I will not let the nerve, energy, and blood to flow through me properly.

I AM THE ANKLE

Throughout your life I have supported your weight and given flexibility to your steps. If I am strong, you take strong, flexible steps in life, and are able to twist and turn at a moment's notice. My joint is filled with fluid and provides a cushion to absorb some of the impact of walking and running.

I am, however, far more important than that. The front and outside of me is controlled primarily by the liver and gall bladder meridians, which are the primary energy systems involved with planning and decision making. The liver (being yin in nature) plans my biochemical makeup and helps to plan my life. Its partner, the gall bladder (being yang in nature), then makes the final decision and acts.

The stomach and spleen/pancreas control the inside of me. They energetically represent the conscious and subconscious mind, respectively. The process of thinking through and worrying about a subject occurs here.

Now, picture a situation where you have to take a 'step' in life — get married; change job; buy a house; accept a new sporting contract; decide on what school you will attend or career you will follow. Each of these events has to be processed by the bodymind. You think and worry, then finally plan and decide. This process goes on in many aspects of your body but the energic processing of it occurs in me as you move around on me. This local movement helps to activate the whole process. The stronger, healthier, and more flexible I am, the easier the whole thinking/deciding process occurs.

If you take too long to make your decision and go through an endless cycle of worrying, deciding, and changing your mind, then you will need me to be extra strong. If I am not very strong and resilient, then I become weaker and prone to injury. You 'sprain your ankle' and when I swell, the energy and fluids increase in me and I lose my flexibility. This will often force you to make your decision.

If you maintain this worrying/indecisive habit pattern over a long period of time, then I will become progressively weak. Eventually, to counteract this my master, the brain, will 'strengthen' me by making me more rigid. You will give this rigidity the label of 'arthritis.'

The illustrations I have given with the four joints of the legs and arms are only a simple version. I hope they have given you an appreciation of the inner workings of the energy systems of the bodymind. Remember that there are many other factors that can be involved. For example, the elbow and wrist are connected by the muscles between them. Those muscles also have their own story to tell that will strongly influence the health of the elbow and wrist. Further, the arm is influenced by the shoulder joint and the muscles around it. That is yet another story.

The study of all this is fascinating. If you really understand the energic psychological makeup of the body, you will then start to appreciate how disease really develops and is maintained.

Fortunately, you do not have to understand all this to be able to effectively treat the related conditions with BodyTalk. With BodyTalk, we show the brain and heart what is wrong and link them clearly to the problem. The brain brings about the changes that are necessary and they are then synthesized in the heart.

The bodymind knows best how to treat itself. Any interference by other people is only a compromise for the real power of healing that lies innate within our systems.

Body Chemistry

S A L I V A
- *Treating viruses, infections, parasites, food intolerances, accumulated toxins, and allergies;*
- Linking them to the rest of the system and emotions where necessary

This is the original treatment that started BodyTalk. In my six-year search for a cure for a chronic virus in my system, I finally met someone who had the original version of this treatment. It worked spectacularly in three days and launched me into a study of the principles used and the eventual development of the system now known as BodyTalk.

With this treatment the BodyTalk practitioner can, under the direction of the body, effectively eliminate chronic and acute viruses, infections, and parasites from the system in a few days. This has very important ramifications in health care because viruses have long been an elusive target for medicine and the treatment for parasites often feels worse than the complaint.

This treatment also eliminates allergies, food intolerances and toxins, quickly enabling people to live normal lives. If the body is correctly balanced, you can eat what you like in the vast majority of cases. There are the occasional patients that do not respond fully, but even they notice increased tolerance and reduction of symptom intensity.

This treatment is so simple and yet so critically important. It will be covered in detail and taught later in this book.

Emotional

PRESENT

- Heart (self-esteem, love issues)
- Pelvis (sensuality and sexuality issues)
- Body image, body acceptance
- Relationships
- Current life situations

PAST

- Lifetime periods (specific years in the life)
- Past relationships (mother, father, family, others)
- Childbirth, fetal life
- Specific incidents and events
- Specific fears and phobias

SPECIFIC

- Treating of the emotion behind one of the specific physical imbalances or body parts
- Treating the emotion behind specific injuries
- Treating the emotion behind specific diseases, food intolerances, and allergies

Since I will not be covering this treatment in this book, I will explain the extremely important role of emotions in disease in some detail now. Whenever the other basic BodyTalk treatments for different conditions are not responding fully, in most cases it is because there are active emotions involved that are contributing to the disease process. For example, many food intolerances will not clear until the emotional relationship with the intolerance is corrected.

Memory can be stored actively or passively in the bodymind. When the memory is passive, we remember and store experiences as simple memory traces in the mind. The stronger or more interesting the memories, the easier it is to recall them. Passive memory is a healthy normal function of the body and the desirable situation.

Active memory is a state where we store the memory with an emotional charge. This occurs when we haven't fully synthesized the emotional content of the experience. Our body then stores the emotion in the fascia of the muscles or connective tissue at a location in concordance with the bioenergetic nature of the body. For example, fear relates to the kidney meridian which, in turn, relates to several muscles and areas of the body. An unsynthesized fearful experience, therefore, will be stored in one of those related areas. In the case of fear (kidneys) it could be the psoas muscle or the ligaments around the knee.

An example of this would be a car accident. Two scenarios can occur:

- The person may synthesize their emotions and fully recover;
- A person may have a car accident that was very traumatic and, because of various factors going on at the time, never had a chance to fully synthesize the emotional associations

Ten years later the person in case one can recall or talk about their accident as a simple description of an event that was traumatic in their life but is now only a memory.

The second scenario is very different. In this case, the person will be emotionally traumatized by the recall of the accident. When talking about it, they may still experience fear, anxiety, grief, anger, or whatever emotions were involved at

71

the time. In other words, their memory is active and associated with stored emotional trauma. When the thought process of the accident is initiated, the brain links the thought to the stored emotion.

Whenever this happens the body is stressed, especially in any areas associated with the accident.

For example, they may have injured their knee in the accident. Whenever the trauma is reactivated, the knee may undergo pathological change inducing pain and discomfort in the weeks thereafter.

In more serious scenarios, the active memory is unconscious. In these cases, the patient's bodymind is not consciously aware of the memory associations. Whenever they see and/or hear about an accident, or even watch one in a movie, their subconscious mind triggers the emotional association, and the person feels anxiety, fear, etc. that they cannot explain in relation to their current circumstances. Furthermore, many symptoms may suddenly flare up (such as the knee mentioned earlier), and they cannot find reasons for the occurrence at that point in their life.

People collect a smorgasbord of active memories in a lifetime that collectively compound any health problem they have. These problems will eventually create health issues in a patient who seems to have no particular reason for getting sick under the circumstances they are enjoying at the time.

The sickness can be mental or physical and may be simply triggered by watching a movie that portrayed an event similar to a painful subconscious memory stored in the patient's bodymind.

A typical case was Jennifer who presented with depression, general aching in the body, fatigue and a feeling of severe body weakness.

By asking her innate wisdom, we established that the physical cause was depleted adrenals and a mild chronic virus. However, it was also established that these were not the primary causes of Jennifer's problems, just the 'symptoms' the body was manifesting to 'explain' the disease.

The primary cause was narrowed down to her childhood abuse. Again, using The BodyTalk System™, we determined that this illness manifested a few days after she watched a movie depicting a father beating his child!

The etiology of the disease was:

- The child was abused and never fully resolved the emotional factors involved even though her relationship with the father was currently

72

'normal'.

- The emotional memory was stored in the body and triggered subconsciously by the scene in the movie. Stressful emotions were released creating physiological changes in the body that weakened the immune system (virus), depressed the heart emotions (depression), and weakened the adrenals (tiredness).
- Because the emotion was trying to emerge and wasn't recognized by the mind, the body diverted it into generalized pain. (Many pains are simply the body's way of diverting focus so that we do not experience emotional trauma.)
- The physical treatment of the symptoms could have given the patient a temporary reprieve. Many times, however, the symptoms do not disappear fully and/or they return quickly, unless the original emotional trauma is resolved.
- By using The BodyTalk Emotional Synthesis Therapy (EST), we were able to disconnect the link between the brain and the stored active emotional memory. An emotion will only be stored when it is 'fed' by underlying thought patterns. Once you cut off the supply of thought from the brain, the emotion loses its support system and dissolves.
- Once the emotional basis was cleared, the patient recovered fully in about three days.

The BodyTalk EST System is very simple. Because it works at the level of the subconscious mind, the patient does not even need to remember the specific emotional traumas. Once isolated, the BodyTalk treatment involves connecting three trigger points on the head with the fingers, doing specific eye movements, and tapping the head and sternum lightly to cause the brain to disassociate from the active memory. The process takes around two minutes and often only one treatment is required to clear an active memory and bring about lasting health changes on the physical and mental/emotional levels.

In another case, Pam suffered severe recurring headaches over a period of about four months. She would often have them three or four times a week. Chiropractic care helped significantly because they seemed to stem from tension in her neck and jaw.

The innate wisdom was consulted and it was determined that the primary problem was emotional—to do with her relationship with her daughter. It was traced back to strong guilt feelings. When she was pregnant with her daughter, she was having enormous financial burdens and a strained relationship with her husband. He was angry that she was pregnant because of the burden it would place on them. In desperation she attempted a home abortion. It was unsuccessful and she ended up having the child and derived great joy from her.

Deep down, however, the subconscious guilt she felt was enormous. I asked why she started manifesting the headaches now? The answer was simple. Her daughter was now six months pregnant and having relationship problems with her husband. The tension in the neck and jaw was triggered when the daughter announced her pregnancy five months earlier.

The triggering occurred subconsciously. Once the memory was activated and the traumatic emotional content dissolved using BodyTalk, the neck and jaw tension—and associated headaches—disappeared permanently overnight. She later recalled that every headache started after a conversation with her daughter, although she didn't make the connection at the time.

Another case involved Mark, who had a multitude of food intolerances. He had a list of foods that upset his digestive system and triggered many allergic responses in him. The problems started in his early twenties; Mark was now thirty-two.

His case was emotionally-based and associated with his early childhood. With help from the BodyTalk feedback, he recalled many fights with his parents over food. Often it was because he didn't want to eat certain foods and he was reminded of the 'starving children in Africa'. Other times it was simply that most of the fights his parent's had took place at the dinner table while he was eating. He was a sensitive boy and the collective associations of emotional trauma and food created an active emotional memory in his system.

The food intolerances became very noticeable in his early twenties because that was when he married and started a family. He suddenly found himself in battle with his own child over food. A subconscious link to the stored active emotional memory occurred and he rapidly developed eating disorders and food intolerance. The BodyTalk emotional treatment cleared the active emotional memory stored in his body and the food intolerance all cleared within two weeks.

The incredible thing about The BodyTalk System™ of treating active emotional storage is that it does not require psychological therapy, extensive treatment, or intense emotional discomfort. The traumatic memory can be cleared without the practitioner needing to know the details of the event.

There are times when the patient may recall an event they would really prefer not to relate. In these cases, it is sufficient for the patient to reflect on the event while being treated. Nothing has to be said or explained.

In other cases, the memory may be so traumatic that the mind refuses to recall it. Good results in these cases are still obtained by locating the time of the trauma (e.g. age sixteen), and then treating while the patient is reflecting on being sixteen. The technique seems to trigger the subconscious mind into clearing the active emotion without it having to surface as a painful memory. The limitation here is that it may take several treatments to clear, compared to the one treatment for specifically-recalled events.

Not all active emotional factors are related to specific events or accumulated experiences. There are many emotional triggers that are initiated by learned attitudes and belief systems. For example, a person may have been brought up in a household where racial prejudice existed against a particular section of society. (e.g. blacks, Mexicans, Jews, whites, etc.) If this was the case, then a negative emotional association may occur. He/she may have been told ridiculous stories as a child of Mexicans being violent and treacherous. This attitude becomes a 'belief' that is associated with emotions of fear and anxiety. A belief is really an expectation, or assumption, that something will happen. If you have the belief that Mexicans are violent, there will be an associated expectation or assumption of violence when meeting a Mexican.

As an adult, you may pride yourself on having transcended your prejudiced upbringing and now feel that you are no longer part of that ignorant past culture. However, you may find that you have recently developed numerous stress related health problems. You eat well, exercise, meditate, and have a happy life, yet here you are with all these anxiety symptoms.

Through therapies such as BodyTalk or the Breakthrough system, you may discover that your symptoms are rooted in a stored active emotion because of a belief system. Eventually, you realize that your symptoms started a week after a new Mexican employee started working with you.

Deep down the active emotional trigger still exists as a belief system embedded in your subconscious. Proximity to a Mexican triggered all those anxieties the little boy felt, even though you consciously liked the person. The BodyTalk System™ would clear that link between the negative belief system and the stored anxiety. In turn, this would not only clear the disease but, once and for all, eliminate the negative belief.

The bodymind is an incredibly complex system of mental, emotional, and physical dynamic interaction. At last, techniques such as The BodyTalk System™ provide effective ways to simplify those interactions and reduce the negative elements quickly and permanently.

We often read articles where psychologists criticize health care practitioners who treat emotional disorders when they are not trained in classical psychology. When you consider that most diseases have an emotional component and will not respond fully until this emotional component is synthesized, does this mean that no heath care practitioner should treat disease—only psychologists? Surely psychologists are not suggesting that emotional health and physical disease are not intimately interwoven and must not be addressed concurrently!

BodyTalk is providing a safe approach to handling this important situation. Whenever the emotional condition is serious enough to merit the specialized help of psychologists, then the innate wisdom of the body will clearly indicate it. I have sent several patients to psychiatrists because they needed the more specialized care.

What Disorders Can BodyTalk Help?

MODULE TWO

Cellular Repair

- Vaccines (damage caused by vaccines);
- Hereditary genetics (treatment of aspects of hereditary genetic diseases where possible);
- Accumulated cellular destruction (repairing the damage caused during the lifetime by various chemical, physical, or emotional traumas)

This is one of the newer developments of BodyTalk and I am still discovering the extent of its potential. Originally the technique was developed to help the body recover from damage caused by vaccines. Many mothers are aware that problems have developed in their children subsequent to a childhood vaccination. Not all children are affected but the percentage is disturbingly high. It appears that some children have an allergic reaction to the base product that the vaccine was cultured on. For example, some vaccines are cultured on egg. If the child had an intolerance to egg, then an allergic reaction will set in, weakening the immune system when the body is exposed to the vaccine. This seems to leave the immune system damaged and the child then develops many food intolerances and allergies. In turn, these allergies affect the child's mood, attention span, and general health.

With this technique the BodyTalk practitioner seems to be able to repair the damage. Naturally, this also affects adults and is more widespread than authorities wish to admit.

While using this technique I discovered that it was also affecting many other aspects of cell damage including apparent genetic weaknesses. Several cases of supposed hereditary disorders have responded to this treatment. The results have been very encouraging and I look forward to further research into this important area.

CASE HISTORY:

Susan had a long history of a weakened immune system. She seemed to constantly catch everything that was going around and blood tests showed that she had chronic viruses in her system. There were major endocrine disruptions and she was diagnosed with severe Chronic Fatigue Syndrome.

Her innate wisdom told me that her problem started with a vaccination at age 13 years. She immediately started crying because she vividly remembered what happened and the years of being told by doctors that it was coincidence. At the time, she lived in South Carolina when there was a 'swine flu' scare. Hundreds were vaccinated and many, like Susan, ended up in hospital with what appeared to be a series of infections. She was assured that it was not swine flu and the timing was coincidental! She knew her illnesses started with that vaccination.

Once I did the cell repair treatment, her road to health was swift. Susan now enjoys a healthy, normal immune system.

Extrinsic Balancing: The Reciprocals

UPPER BODY / LOWER BODY

- upper shoulder/iliac crest
- shoulder tip/hip
- shoulder front/front of hip
- shoulder back/back of hip
- elbow/knee
- wrist/ankle
- navel/coccyx

HEAD / BODY

- vomer/xiphoid
- temporal bone/innominate bone
- zygoma/pubic crest
- mouth/navel
- ear/axilla
- eye/breast

HEAD / SPINAL COMPLEX

- TMJ/sacroiliac joint
- sphenoid/coccyx
- occiput/sacrum
- styloid/lumbosacral
- upper spine/lower spine

There are two major system concepts I deal with in this section of BodyTalk and, as they are arbitrary divisions within an indivisible complex, they will be loosely referred to as the *extrinsic* and *intrinsic* systems.

The extrinsic system refers to the surface energy of the body which encompasses such concepts as the *Wei* (protective) energy of Chinese medicine and the protective and synthesizing aspect of the electromagnetic field around the body talked about in modern bioenergetics.

The intrinsic system relates to the internal communication along the connective tissue and fascia of the body. It is in this system that we store the memory and emotions of the body. A more detailed discussion will be covered later.

At this stage we are concerned with the extrinsic system with regard to one of its main functions. Namely, to provide a rapid form of communication between the various parts of the body.

This communication is more rapid than the slower nerve fibers and meridians. This extrinsic energy:

- Flows just above the skin, on the surface, and just underneath it.
- It provides a network of communication that has loose and more versatile pathways than its slower and more confined cousins within the body.

The energy communicates with the brain through the skull and has major entrance and exit points all over the body—particularly at joints.

These points usually work in pairs and seem to mimic the 'circuit breakers' of an electrical system. As pairs, they are usually on *opposite sides of the body at opposite ends*.

For example, the right knee and left elbow; the left hip and right shoulder, etc. They are called the *reciprocal pairs.*

In this section of BodyTalk we test the integrity of these 'circuit breakers' and, if faulty, treat them. Clinically, this appears to correct faulty communication within the body and encourages significant healing.

A simple concept is to envisage a situation where the system has been overloaded by stress or disease, and one of these 'circuit breakers' has 'blown'. This compels the body to function using an inferior backup circuit until the crisis is over. In many cases, the patient never fully recovers or the system, due to various stress factors, is unable to restore the integrity of the 'circuit breaker' in question. The system persistently malfunctions and the patient's body continues to 'do it the hard way' at the expense of health.

Since the general health of the bodymind system is totally dependent on good communication, the importance of healthy 'circuit breakers' cannot be underestimated. The bodymind must literally be able to talk to itself. We restore that communication—hence the name BodyTalk!

The restoration of all the malfunctioning 'circuit breakers' using The BodyTalk System™:

- Significantly affects the total health of the patient;
- Boosts the general energy levels of the patient;
- Lifts the patient's mood and strengthens resolve. (Possibly a side affect of the general energy boost);
- Goes a long way toward balancing the energy meridian system;
- Has a dramatic effect on the overall structural integrity of the patient.

(Significant changes in posture are noticeable to the trained eye);

- Improves total circulation and lymphatic drainage of the body. (Probably due to the postural changes);
- Improves the total breathing cycle;
- Reduces total muscle tension in the body. (Again the posture);
- Greatly improves the digestive system. (A mixture of the above factors along with the improved communication within the bodymind complex);
- Balances out the function of the nervous system. (Evident by the clinical results in many neurological conditions);
- Clinically, it appears that the effect of correcting a 'circuit breaker' is not necessarily local. For example, the elbow/knee connection, when corrected, does not necessarily correct an arthritic knee problem. The ramifications seem more far-reaching. These techniques are used to balance the general musculature and skeleton of the body. By linking the reciprocal points of the body which are found on opposite sides and opposite ends of the body, the BodyTalk practitioner can stimulate the brain into rebalancing the mechanical systems of the body to restore normal function. This has direct ramifications on spinal problems, arthritis, and chronic and acute injuries.

Bodyworkers also note that the structure of the body has a large influence on the function. Correction of the reciprocal will also have significant effect on the physiology of the body.

CASE HISTORY:

Pam was thirty years old and had advanced rotatory scoliosis (curvature of the spine). This condition was extremely debilitating and kept her in constant pain. She had limited range of movement in her body and even walking and standing was difficult.

The balancing of her reciprocal segments dramatically changed the way the body adapted to the condition. Over the next six months Pam had increasing movement, reduction of pain, and general feeling of muscular strength.

One year later Pam was able to walk and stand for long periods without pain and had taken up beach volleyball. Her shoulders and scapular were more even, her pelvis was straighter, and the curvature less pronounced.

Lymphatic

- Linking the zygoma to the lymph glands of the neck, sub-clavicular area, breast, splenic sub diaphragm area, abdomen, groin;
- Specific lymphatic drainage massages where necessary.

In many people the lymph system has become dangerously sluggish and it needs to be 'spring cleaned.' Very often the lymph ducts become blocked and the lymph just accumulates in the tissues. This means that the waste products are not eliminated from the cells effectively and the cells will start malfunctioning. This will also set up a breeding ground for infection and local decay of the cells.

This is particularly important in women in the pelvis. When the lymphatic system becomes sluggish, the circulation of estrogen is impaired and the reproductive system does not drain properly. Common symptoms are pelvic congestion and endometriosis, ovarian cysts and ovarian malfunction, period pain, irregular and abnormal periods, the formation of adhesions around the uterus that can lead to painful sex and bowel irritations.

When the lymphatic drainage of the diaphragm is impaired, the lungs and heart will drain poorly leading to chronic lung weaknesses and congestion of the heart.

Once the major lymph ducts have become impaired, the whole lymphatic system is compromised and circulation throughout the body is reduced and sluggish. Fluid accumulates and the health deteriorates.

The BodyTalk System™ provides a simple procedure to induce the body to clear the lymphatic system.

CASE HISTORY:

Jan had history of breast swelling and tenderness in the period between ovulation and her menstrual flow, which was also painful and heavy. Eventually, she noticed the formation of enlarged lymph nodes. Her medical checks determined that they were not malignant but the doctor suggested removing them as a precaution. He explained that this would simply remove the lumps but not solve her problem with swelling and tenderness.

The BodyTalk System found linkage problems between her pituitary gland and ovaries; adrenals and ovaries; liver and uterus. The BodyTalk lymphatic technique was also used. The lumps disappeared in nine days, her next menstrual cycle improved a little with the breast tenderness and period pain. The following month, after a second BodyTalk treatment, all symptoms disappeared.

The Nervous and Circulatory Systems

- Linking the brain to the body parts, organs, and endocrines for nerve flow to, or within, the part;
- Linking the heart (circulation) to the body parts, organs, and endocrines for blood flow to, or within, the part

The first item links the brain and central nervous system to the various body parts. The link to Western medical concepts and chiropractic are obvious since it is well established that the nervous system is vital to the functioning of the body. These links help promote correct nerve flow and balance to all the parts of the body.

The second item involves linking the circulation to the various body parts to promote blood flow to an organ, endocrine, or body part. This dramatically improves the circulation and vital function of any part involved. Many cases of poor circulation to areas such as the hands and feet have effectively restored the circulation in one or two treatments.

Energy Systems

LINKING THE SEVEN CHAKRAS

The linking of the seven chakras and what they can do is covered in detail later in this book.

VIVAXIS

Vivaxis is also covered in this book in detail. Briefly, the vivaxis technique is designed to reorient the body to its surroundings. Many people are found to be out of synch with the energy fields surrounding them, e.g. the magnetic fields of the earth. It seems to primarily affect those who have moved from their birth place into new energy fields that they were not able to adapt to. The main effect of vivaxis disorientation seems to be the holding of chronic disease in the body and homesickness! It does seem to help in 'jet lag' as well as helping people to settle into a new home or environment.

> ### CASE HISTORY:
> *Ann had a history of fibromyalgia that was unresponsive to the many heath care systems she had tried. She mentioned that although she had been living in Australia for 23 years and had all her family there, she was always homesick for England and felt like a 'fish out of water' where she lived.*
>
> *When the vivaxis correction was made, the homesickness disappeared, never to return. Further, she started responding positively to her treatments.*

MERIDIANS AND SUGAR BALANCES

- Balance the 12 meridian pulses
- Balance the sugar pulses (liver, adrenals, pancreas)
- *The pancreas reflex point*

These techniques enable the BodyTalk practitioner to balance the meridians of the body according to the priority set by the body. It only takes a few minutes and can have dramatic affect on the whole bodymind system. The effect of balancing the meridians is well documented in acupuncture, which achieves the same thing only with needles.

Musculo-skeletal

- Intrinsic treatment of the fascia for each of the body parts indicated;
- Treatment of specific sports injuries and arthritic joints

I could write a separate book about this section because it covers so much territory. In this section the BodyTalk practitioner is treating the deep fascia, muscles, and bones of the body for arthritis, muscular disorders, joint pathologies, bruises, cuts, sprains, sports injuries, and rehabilitation.

A very simple treatment system is applied so that the techniques can be mastered quickly. The key lies in the linking of parts. If the ankle is injured, the innate wisdom is asked, through muscle testing, to what to link the ankle. Sometimes it will be to its reciprocal partner, the wrist on the opposite side. Other times it will be to an organ, endocrine, body tissue, section of the brain, or an emotional link. Remember the relationship of the emotions to the joints discussed earlier. Once all the links are reestablished, the ankle will repair much faster than normal and more completely.

In BodyTalk, I have found that most injuries have linkages to stress and emotions that predisposed the patient to injuring that area in the first place. For example, if the patient is trying to take a major step in their life and having difficulty in making the decision, then they are going to be susceptible to injuring their ankle. Once the injury occurs, the ankle will be best treated by linking it to the organs related to decisions (gall bladder) and worry (pancreas) as well as to any active memory related to the decision. The person may be contemplating a second marriage with active memories of a disastrous first marriage. These memories are retarding the decision making process and creating stress in the area of the ankle. The injury is then inevitable.

If normal therapy is used to help the injury, the ankle often will have complications and slow recovery. The patient will often re-injure the area or its reciprocal, the wrist. The BodyTalk System™ utilizes the deep inner-knowing of the patient to ensure the underlying factors and mechanical injury are fully treated. This is true healing and must certainly point to the type of healing approach we are heading toward in the 21st century.

Environmental

- Checking for links between the patient and factors in his/her environment; environmental factors include people, animals, chemicals, physical objects, and stressful situations;
- Linking the physical body to the environment;
- Linking the emotions to the environment

Environment is a vital area of BodyTalk. Up to now we have been establishing relationship problems within the bodymind complex and linking them to bring about synchronicity and harmony. We must remember, however, that the bodymind complex is also part of an even bigger environmental complex—the world—that also has interrelationships and needs synchronicity in order for each part to function well. Very often, the practitioner will find that the body will not fully heal until unresolved conflicts with factors and people within the patient's environment are linked and harmonized.

Our bodymind is in a dynamic systems relationship with the people around us, the objects, chemicals, etc. The BodyTalk practitioner can establish what is going wrong with all those factors and what to do about it. Time and again I have seen people who have had good therapy but not fully respond because their system was not harmonized and synchronized to their immediate environment.

CASE HISTORY:

Seven-year-old John had mild asthma and many allergies. His lungs were weak and he easily caught infections. He had been receiving acupuncture and homeopathy with significant improvement but once he stopped the regular treatments his condition returned.

There were many links to restore in John's body and his immune system had to be repaired from the effects of vaccines he had received. However, the big change occurred when he was tested to his environment. He tested weak to his mother who was a concerned, loving, but overprotective person. He showed that his mother 'smothered' his lungs and this stressed his adrenals. After I did the correction, his breathing improved immediately, color came back into his cheeks within ten minutes, and he felt and looked very different.

CASE HISTORY:

Norm had been suffering from severe headaches for nine months. The BodyTalk treatment protocol took me straight to environmental factors. It was not people, but an object. We narrowed it down to his car. Norm then realized that his headaches always came on after he had been driving the car. He was also aware that driving recently had become traumatic to him.

Further questioning established that he had been in a car accident a year ago in which he was hurt quite badly. The car he now drove was the very same car he had the accident in. It became clear that he had an active memory around the car. It could hurt him badly.

Norm was treated to the car and the active memory was disassociated using the BodyTalk emotional treatment. His headaches stopped immediately and he was still able to drive the same car.

In the last two chapters you have been given a glimpse of the scope of BodyTalk. In the next chapters you will be taught some of the techniques that are easy to learn and very safe to use. I urge you to try them yourselves and discover the magic of BodyTalk. Learn how health care can—and should—be in the coming years.

I should warn you that you will not always obtain great results with the few techniques you learn. For example, the treatment for allergies can be spectacular but sometimes it will not hold for long because there are other underlying factors around the allergy for which care needs to be taken. The most common factors would be the emotional components. In these cases you should look for help from a BodyTalk practitioner who knows the whole system, or your local health care practitioner.

The techniques on the following pages can transform your life. I have received much e-mail from excited people who had learned a few simple techniques from my web site and dramatically helped members of their family or friends. In the meantime, I hope the book will inspire many of you to train as BodyTalk practitioners and help make this world a safer and healthier place to live.

The SB Technique

THE INITIALS SB STAND FOR SPHENO-BASILAR. THIS REFERS TO A PART OF the skull that is often wrongly referred to as a joint. It is the cartilaginous junction of the sphenoid and basal bones of the skull and it is mobile in healthy people.

We are interested in this joint because it has an important role in the breathing cycle and the function of the pituitary gland.

As we breathe in and out, the SB joint moves up and down in synchronicity with the breathing. This very small movement affects the circulation in the brain, the function of the pituitary gland, the master gland of the endocrine system, and the breathing cycles. (It should be noted that there are two different rhythms to which the skull moves. One is the breathing cycle and the other is the cranial pulse described in cranio-sacral therapy. The cranial pulse is different than the breathing cycle and is superimposed upon the basic breathing cycle. The brain has very complex patterns of movements that reflect the complexity of its functions.)

If the movement of the SB is compromised, it will affect the brain and general function of the body profoundly. There are many factors that can restrict the movement of this juncture.

One common factor is when blows to the head at just the wrong angle restrict it. You can hit yourself on the head many times and do no damage. However, if you hit your head in the exact wrong position at the wrong angle, then severe problems can evolve. A typical example would be arising from a squatting position and hitting yourself on the top of the head. If the blow is exactly on the suture near the front of the head that separates the frontal bone and the two parietal bones, then this blow will profoundly damage the SB movement. A fraction of an inch either way and no harm is done!

Another cause for SB locking is emotional. If, as a child, you spent a lot of time in a startled reflex, living in fear of punishment, then this will create long-term locking. The scenario would be four-year-old Peter raiding the cupboard for sweets. Suddenly his father's booming voice yells, "What are you doing?" Peter has a startled reflex, causing him to inhale suddenly and hold his breath. If this is done repetitively through similar situations and there is definite stored fear of the consequences, the SB will jam in a 'locked up' position in a way that Peter will always tend to breathe in but not breathe out fully. The act of breathing out is the act of fully letting go. Peter will learn not to let go in life because he believes he can get into trouble suddenly at any time. He will develop a defensive personality, be hyperactive, unable to relax, and emotionally uptight. This will continue to influence his health and every aspect of his life even in adulthood.

In the opposite scenario, a football player may be kneed in the head exactly on the suture mentioned earlier. This causes the SB to be 'locked down' and the football player never fully recovers. He cannot breathe in fully and breathes out too easily and too far. He develops a depressed attitude to life and looses the 'spark' that made him a great athlete. His body will under function and he will feel like he has to drag himself around.

These are extreme examples. Most of us fit somewhere in between. Some are actually 'locked' both ways and share a little of both symptoms! Minor restrictions of the movement of the SB joint also occur in stress reactions to life and are covered in more detail later. The pituitary gland sits right over the SB junction and the movement of the SB is what contributes to the circulation within the pituitary. This circulation is vital for pituitary function. The pituitary is often referred to as the master gland of the endocrine system and problems with the pituitary can have ramifications throughout the body with a multitude of hormonal symptoms.

The BodyTalk practitioner is particularly interested in establishing a free SB juncture because of its effect on breathing. You will remember from an earlier chapter that BodyTalk relies heavily on the breathing cycle for the brain to establish what frequencies within the body need correcting. A healthy breathing cycle also contributes greatly to the healing of the body. Yoga says "perfect breath, perfect health."

When a person is breathing fully, the diaphragm moves up and down freely with a good range of motion. This movement of the diaphragm is vital to the functioning of the digestive system. The diaphragm 'massages' the digestive organs and helps to stimulate their functioning. In situations where breathing is restricted, the digestive process is compromised and the person will often have a history of poor digestion, energy deficiency, poor liver metabolism, poor sugar handling, and many more related disorders. Although there are many other causes of digestive disorders, this one should not be overlooked. There is also a specific BodyTalk treatment for the diaphragm covered later in the BodyTalk protocol.

You can now probably see why I want the SB corrected first in a BodyTalk treatment. *In fact, it should be corrected first before any treatment of any modality!* Once the SB is corrected, the brain will have better circulation, the pituitary and endocrine system will function better, and the breathing cycle will have improved. (This can be demonstrated by using a spirometer to measure the breath volume before and after the correction.)

The correction of the SB juncture is very easy.

Before you test for the SB problem, you will need to have trained your patient to the yes/no protocol described in chapter seven. Once this has been established for the patient you are testing, you can move on.

To Test for SB Problems

- Ask the patient to take a deep breath right in and ask, "Is there a problem with the SB?" If the patient tests *yes* (weak), then they have a problem with their SB locked down. (A scenario like the blow to the head.)
- Then ask the patient to breathe all the way out—right out, as far as possible. Ask "is there a problem with SB?" If the patient tests *yes* (weak), then they have a problem with the SB locked up. (The typical startled child reflex.)

As I said before, some people will test weak both ways. Some will be just a bit weak, others very weak, often indicating a big problem.

91

The treatment is exactly the same for both scenarios. It doesn't matter which way they went weak (or both ways), the treatment will correct everything. Remember that you can't do any harm with BodyTalk. If the patient did not have a SB problem and you treated it, nothing would happen, *you would not do any harm.*

To Treat SB Problems

- Have the patient place their index finger inside their mouth so that they are touching the hard palate (roof of the mouth) almost as far back as the start of the soft palate.
- Place your finger on the pituitary spot, which is the bridge of the nose where the nose joins the forehead.
- With both these contacts being held, use your spare hand to tap the head and sternum while the patient is asked to take two full deep breaths.

The tapping can be done so that the head is tapped for one of the breaths and the sternum for the other breath. Some practitioners get bored with that and prefer to alternate every few seconds between the head and sternum. Either way works just fine. Just remember to make sure your fingers are spread when tapping the head to ensure that you are covering both sides of the midline front to back.

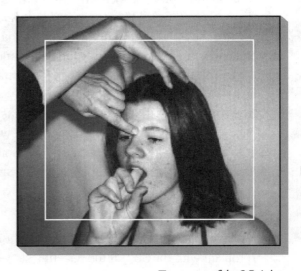

Treatment of the S.B. Joint

Retest

Make sure that the treatment has worked by doing the test again. This time the answer to the question, "Is there a problem with the SB?" will be no.

Most of the BodyTalk treatments are that easy. You may at first have some problems with the muscle test and feel that you are not sure. This is normal. It will take a while to develop the skills and you may have a patient who is not too cooperative or 'aware' when you first set out. No one is that keen on being practiced upon by an amateur. This will change quickly, especially when the results start flowing.

CASE HISTORY:

Vin was 35 years old and felt 50 years old. There was no particular symptom worrying him that he could actually complain about. He had simply felt slowed down, lethargic, and dull minded for years. He was a good social tennis player and even his game had lost its edge. It seemed like he had lost his coordination. Perhaps his greatest complaint was feeling foggy headed, and although his gardening job was not intellectually demanding, he was very aware of loosing his confidence in his ability to hold his own with his children in computer games and other activities.

Immediately after tapping out the SB juncture, Vin said he felt his head clearing. This continued over the next few days. Later in the BodyTalk treatment I asked his innate wisdom when his problems had started and it quite clearly narrowed it down to an accident he had eight years earlier. A box had fallen from a high shelf onto the top of his head. He remembered it because the doctor said he had concussion and he could not go to an important baseball game he wanted to see.

Although he recovered from the concussion, it was obvious that his SB had been jammed down and all his symptoms developed progressively from that point in time. When I saw him for a follow up one month later, it was like talking to a different person. There was a glint in the eye and a sense of presence and clarity that was missing before.

In most cases it is difficult to say that one particular treatment helps any particular symptom because the BodyTalk practitioner will always be doing a collection of techniques according to the demands of the innate wisdom of the patient. Obviously, based on what I have been saying in the first few chapters, all the techniques are of equal importance because of the dynamic laws of synchronicity within the body. As in a hologram, each part reflects the whole.

For the rest of this book I will continue to give case histories at the end of a technique as a means of explaining the possible ramifications of a treatment. I will assume that you will keep in mind that each technique will have been performed in conjunction with others.

There are no formulas in BodyTalk. At no stage do I teach how to help specific conditions. When students ask, "How do I treat bronchitis, or arthritis of the knee, or a bowel infection?" My answer is always the same. Do the full treatment protocol and ask the innate wisdom of the body what to do. Every single case will be different.

Naturally, you are not learning the whole treatment protocol in this book. The techniques I am teaching you combine safely to help many conditions. The difference is that without the knowledge of the full BodyTalk protocol you may not have results as quickly. In some cases the results will be limited or not happen at all. In these cases you need to refer to a BodyTalk practitioner or other health care practitioner.

The wonderful thing is that, provided you always ask, "Is there a problem with ...?" before you treat, *you will do no harm.*

CHAPTER

12

Vivaxis

THE VIVAXIS TECHNIQUE HAS BEEN AROUND FOR A LONG TIME. I FIRST learned the procedure in 1976, long before the evolution of BodyTalk. It is interesting to note that the treatment is still much the same. The technique involved the tapping of the head, way back in 1976. The BodyTalk protocol has added the heart (sternum) tapping to hold and store the changes. Obviously, the original vivaxis treatment was a pointer to the future, only I didn't associate it until 1994.

The vivaxis technique has been clinically effective for many years although the theoretical explanation for exactly what we are doing is still controversial. It appears that there are two main explanations—and possibly both are right—since both account for different results in different cases.

The Birth Vivaxis Theory

This theory says that in our mother's womb we are energetically protected from external influences and energy fields. As a fetus, we have our hereditary genes, and basic physical structure is already determined.

When we are born we are suddenly exposed to the world around us and the energy fields bombarding that particular space. This has the effect of 'stamping' us with a superimposed energy 'blueprint' that will influence many aspects of our physical health and psychological makeup.

Astrologers would see this as the astrological foundation that makes us a Libra or a Virgo, etc. They have long insisted that the exact time and location of our birth determines this and there is a lot of evidence in research to support this. As mentioned before, I am only theorizing here and none of this affects the clinical results other than to give an explanation for some of the symptoms of vivaxis that are described later.

The theory goes on to say that there is a vivaxis (life-axis) formed at the exact location of the birth that continues to stay in that exact location for the rest of our lives. It is well known in physics that many millions of frequencies can stay in the same space without interference. Obviously, in the delivery room of a maternity hospital there would be many vivaxes. I have spoken to 'sensitives' who say they are aware of them.

As we go about life, the vivaxis continues to keep a connection to us by 'transmitting' through the top of our heads. This transmission keeps us up to date with the energy (or planetary?) influences that are affecting us and contributes to our general well-being.

Whenever the transmission is interrupted, problems can occur. This can happen when a person has moved far from home and interference patterns have been set up in the pathway between him and his vivaxis.

For example, it is generally considered that the incidence of vivaxis problems is growing fast. It appears to be a modern problem. There is speculation that the interference is occurring through the existence of nuclear reactors, higher powered electricity grids, and other high energy vortexes that can affect energy transmission of a more subtle nature.

Why does this theory seem to have some credence? One of the main observations of vivaxis is that the majority of sufferers are living a long way from their birth place. A common symptom is unexplained homesickness even when their current abode is home to them. The following case study is typical.

CASE HISTORY:

Gail was a 50 year old English woman who had been living in Australia for thirty years. She was seeing me for chronic arthritis and headaches, but had a slow response to treatment. At the time I was treating her with acupuncture and chiropractic (before my BodyTalk days.) During one of her treatments she half jokingly said "I sure wish you could treat me for this ridiculous homesickness I suffer from constantly." I took her seriously and asked her to explain.

Gail said that she had lived in Australia all these years and loved it. Her children and grandchildren lived here and she considered herself a 'true blue' Aussie. Yet she was constantly aware of this homesickness in the sense that she had a strong desire to go back to England. It was so bad that 14 years previously she and her husband returned to England with possible plans to live there if necessary. They found jobs and stayed there for eight months. During that time her health improved significantly, the homesickness disappeared, and she felt more energized. However, she hated England and the lifestyle there and missed her family. They returned to Australia and her symptoms resurfaced.

The magic words were "unexplained home sickness." She tested very weak for vivaxis and I treated her. A week later she called to say that the homesickness had gone! Subsequently, her response to her treatments for her chronic illnesses improved dramatically.

Key descriptions that often denote vivaxis problems are *chronic, degenerative, stubborn, fatigue, and feeling like a 'fish out of water' as though you do not belong in your environment.*

This leads to the second theory of vivaxis. This theory says that you have a vivaxis problem when you are not aligned with your environment. Your energy patterns are not synchronized with the energy fields around you. This can be within the home, at work, or in the city you live in. It may be a clash with a electrical power grid, overhead power lines, computers, underground streams, and many other variables. Support for this theory comes from the clinical experience of testing people for their vivaxis at my clinic and finding nothing. I then teach the patient to retest themselves (with the help of a friend) at home or work. In the different environment they test positive to the vivaxis. After the vivaxis treatment they notice significant changes in health, moods, or energy within a week or two.

Both theories can seem to apply since one treatment may seem to fix the severe chronic problems—and other factors—that appear to relate to a remote distancing from their place of birth. On other occasions the problem seems to be local.

Testing for Vivaxis

The patient stands with one arm extended at right angles to the body, horizontal to the ground. The practitioner tests the arm by saying, *"Is there a problem with vivaxis?"* If the test is *no* (a strong arm), then the patient rotates to another point of the compass. Usually I have them rotate about 45° at a time. Each location is tested until there is a *yes* answer (the arm is weak). This is the vivaxis weak position. You will find the exact direction by minimizing the degrees of rotation (until now 45°) and retesting until you find the specific direction the patient tests weakest.

Treatment of Vivaxis

With the patient continuing to hold the arm out in that exact position—like an antenna—you will then tap the head and sternum while the patient takes two full breath cycles.

Retest to make sure it is corrected. Then move on and try the rest of the compass circle. I have found that when treating for the remote 'birth' vivaxis, there is usually only one position to correct. However, when treating for local environmental adaptation, there can be several points to treat.

The vivaxis is included in the Essential General Treatments because I have found it to be clinically very important for good general results. Although there are often no specific symptoms as indicators that the vivaxis is needed (for example, many do not feel homesick), I have found that patients who are slow to respond, or even un-responsive to treatment, will often start responding well after correction.

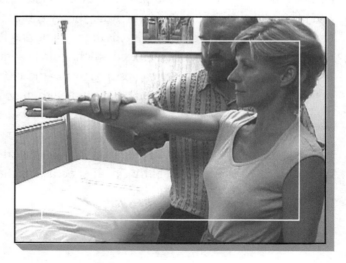

CHAPTER

13

The Basic Cortices

THE UNDERLYING THEORY BEHIND THE CORTICES TREATMENT IS THAT ALL disease is reflected in the brain at some level. In studies on dyslexic children with infra red photography, it was found that there are 'cold' spots of diminished blood supply or cellular activity in the brain cortices on both sides, apparently mirroring each other. When the child has remedial teaching and there are positive improvements in the dyslexia from a clinical perspective, the 'cold' spots had either diminished or gone.

Another study has shown specific cold spots for various mental disorders and other diseases. The theory goes that everything that is going wrong with the body is reflected in the brain as faulty activity. Of course, the question remains, "Which came first, the disease or the brain disturbance?" Under the hologram dynamic interactive theory the question is redundant. It really doesn't matter and we will probably find situations where both concepts are right.

The key is that BodyTalk practitioners are constantly seeing significant improvements in many illness, physical and mental, once these 'cold' spots have been directly 'repaired.' On other occasions it appears that the repair of the brain is only part of the equation and other areas have to be linked for permanent results. I have seen many cases of dyslexia improve dramatically in children—in days—with just the cortex treatment. On other occasions, the innate wisdom asks for complex linkages involving food allergies, spinal problems, endocrine disturbances, and environmental issues before good lasting results are obtained.

What I have found is that the cortices need to be treated on 98% of sick patients as part of their healing process. Sometimes the cortex treatment seems to have little effect at the time but will obviously be an important factor in the total treatment protocol orchestrated by the innate intelligence of the body.

On other occasions I have seen immediate effects that have amazed me as much as the patient.

CASE HISTORY:

Len came for BodyTalk treatment for his digestive problems and skin rash. He had a stroke four years earlier and had lost the use of his right lower arm and hand. After one year of therapy, the specialist said that he would have no improvement and should discontinue therapy.

While I was routinely tapping out his cortices, Len commented that the fingers in his right hand were tingling! I asked him to try to move his fingers. To his amazement, they moved in twitching movements. I continued to keep tapping out his cortices and he felt his hands warming up and many other sensations developing. A week later he return with a 60% range of motion. Over the next few months the muscles in his hand developed and he had near normal use of his hand.

I have seen several stroke cases respond to BodyTalk but most need many links connected. Occasionally, there are conditions where just restoring the brain linkages is enough for significant changes.

The most common 'symptom' of having your cortices tapped out is a subjective increase in wellbeing. People simply feel better in themselves after their cortices have been corrected.

Treating the cortices also appears to have a significant effect on stress levels. I have found that I can send a patient home well balanced after a full treatment and they feel great. That night they have a very stressful incident at home and when they are checked the next day their cortices have 'blown.' Correction of the cortices immediately settles them down and they are calm again. I have taught many patients to use the cortex treatment for stress management. This is not a panacea. It seems to only help short term. Once there is a scenario of long-term stress management problems, the whole BodyTalk treatment protocol needs to be implemented for lasting results. This will particularly involve the correction of the limbic system of the brain.

Treating the cortices is a vital part of the BodyTalk protocol. Because it improves brain function and reduces stress so well, it is essential for all modalities as part of a basic treatment preparation so that the patient can be more responsive to any treatment.

Testing the Basic Cortices

- Run your hand lightly over the head of the patient just brushing the scalp as much as the hair will allow. This action should run from the front of the forehead, right over the head, to the base of the skull.

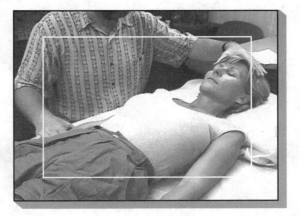

Running the cortices

- When you have done this, ask the body, *"Is there a problem with cortices?"* If the answer is *yes* (weak) then proceed with the treatment.

Treating the Cortices

- Place your hand on the patient's head at the base of the skull and upper neck. While you hold that position, tap the head and sternum, alternating for a full breath cycle.
- Now move your hand up onto the head to the position next to the one you just did. (You are going to systematically cover the whole head.) In the new position, tap out the head and sternum alternating for a full breath.
- This procedure is repeated until you have covered the whole mid-line of the head. It usually takes four positions, although small hands on a big head may take five.
- You now need to cover the side of the head. Have the patient put one

101

hand along the side of the head while you put your hand on the other side. Use your free hand to tap head and sternum, again while the patient takes a full breath.

Once the treatment is completed, retest to confirm the correction.

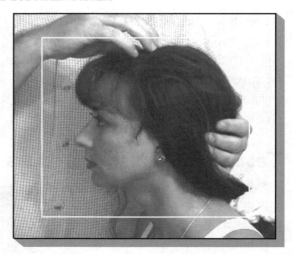

Tapping out the cortices

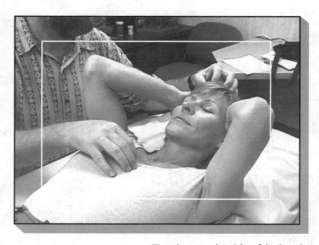

Tapping out the side of the head

Hydration

WATER THERAPY IS OFTEN TALKED ABOUT BUT LITTLE UNDERSTOOD. PEOPLE speak about the importance of water intake and believe 'fluid intake' is based on the supposition that all fluid contains water and therefore all fluids help to supply the water needs of the body. However, coffee, tea, some herb teas, and sodas contain caffeine or caffeine-like substances. Caffeine is a dehydrating agent (diuretic) that increases the function of the kidneys causing dehydration. Therefore, the drinking of these beverages without supplementary pure water has the final effect of dehydrating the tissues and cells.

The water must be taken into the body in its natural form. This can include spring water and clean tap water. Distilled water is controversial because there is an argument that it is 'empty' and will tend to be corrosive to the body in its efforts to dissolve things in itself and leach the body of certain minerals.

Many people seem to think of water as merely a solvent, a packaging material, and means for transportation of other substances in the body. Most emphasis is placed on proteins, minerals, and vitamins. However, water is vital to energy production in the cells, metabolism, and in neurotransmission.

Hydrolysis is the splitting of the water molecule into hydrogen and oxygen. Whenever this occurs, energy is released. The energy produced by water helps to produce ATP—a major source of energy stored in the body.

Many parts of the brain draw much of their energy from water. The brain is 80% water if fully hydrated. Neurotransmission is heavily dependent upon water. The transmission of a nerve occurs via charged minerals called cations. Cation exchange gets its energy from water. Another benefit of water in nerve transmission is the existence of small waterways or micro-streams along the full length of nerves. These float the brain products along microtubules to the nerve ending. When the body is dehydrated, nerve transmission is compromised and brain function is strongly diminished. Chronic nerve pain is often simply the end result of chronic dehydration. Pain in chronic arthritis and similar conditions is often reduced significantly after patient rehydration.

Another important consideration is that water actually holds the cells of the body together. Water keeps the cell membrane together by forming 'hydronium' ions ($H_3O_2^+$) which makes the water 'sticky' and helps bond the cell. This gives the cell a lower viscosity that helps the efficiency of proteins and enzymes. In a dehydrated cell, the metabolism is greatly impaired. This involves all metabolic problems in the body. It has a particularly dramatic effect on sugar metabolism, the immune system, and detoxification.

From a cellular point of view, the transmission of nutrients through the cell wall is conducted by water. Many dehydrated people are malnourished despite excellent diets. Many deficiency conditions are no more than specific dehydration problems.

Dehydration is the greatest producer of free radicals in the body and effective hydration removes free radicals faster than any other therapy. Taking supplements to reduce free radicals is ineffective when the body is dehydrated because they cannot work effectively. Further antioxidant supplements are a waste of money in a fully hydrated body because they are unnecessary!

Lung dehydration is considered a significant factor in respiratory diseases. Sometimes the most dramatic results can be obtained in asthma and chronic bronchitis with simple rehydration.

Dehydration is a major producer of stress in the body and it alters the balance of amino acids. This will allow DNA errors during cell division that can lead to many diseases such as cancer and other cell mutation problems.

Water is also considered a vital conductor of energy such as meridian energy and other body energy systems. When the body is dehydrated, it is very difficult for energy based therapies such as Reiki, polarity therapy, magnetic healing, some aspects of BodyTalk, bioenergetic work, etc., to work. The body simply cannot take full advantage of them. I am finding that the patient who is slower to respond to treatment is invariably dehydrated.

Emotions are synthesized and harmonized by water. Dehydration is a major precursor to emotional and mental disorders. I have yet to test a bipolar (manic-depressive) patient who is not dehydrated. Children, in particular, are very prone to dehydration these days simply because they are not drinking plain water. Hyperactive children are invariably dehydrated and tend to only want to drink liquid in the form of sodas, punches, and other caffeine and sugar-laden beverages.

Dehydration is by far the most important factor in aging. Just look at the skin of the older person. It is simply dehydrated!

Dehydration profoundly affects the movement of lymph through the body and causes the lymph system to clog up and malfunction.

Alcohol dehydrates the body. The morning after headache and aches and pains, can be attributed to the side effects of dehydration. In fact most headaches, including migraine, improve with rehydration.

One of the major problems with hydration therapy up to now has been that many patients who have the symptoms of dehydration will tell you that they drink plenty of water. I have had patients who have come to me for fluid retention because they have far too much fluid in their body. Yet, when I test them for hydration, the test says they are very dehydrated!

The other problem is that drinking large glasses of water often doesn't rehydrate them—it just makes them feel sick. This is like the reaction of the person found in the desert who is given a large amount of water—the body reacts.

It is important to realize that many people have a condition that stops them from having fully hydrated body cells and brain tissue despite their drinking adequate water. The BodyTalk treatment of the cortices of the brain addresses this problem.

The BodyTalk System™ corrects the underlying factors limiting the absorption of water throughout the body. The test and treatment I am showing you is for the general treatment of hydration problems in the body. This will eventually correct the problem throughout the body. BodyTalk practitioners will sometimes need to treat specific stubborn areas to facilitate faster results. For example, they may specifically treat areas like the brain, an arthritic spine, a specific organ such as the liver, or a specific joint such as the knee. In these cases, the effect of the treatment will be faster because it is more specific. Many people notice significant changes in their skin a month or two after treatment as their skin rehydrates and become more youthful in appearance.

Test

- Soak a tissue or cotton bud in some clean water.
- Place the wet tissue to the patient's navel or, if that is hard to get at because of clothing, you can place it over the thymus gland on the sternum.
- You then ask, "Is there a hydration problem?" If the answer is *yes* (weak) then the patient needs treatment.

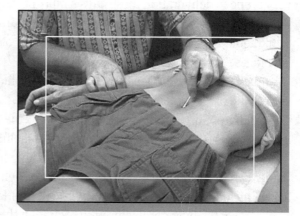

Testing for hydration

Treatment

- Leave the wet tissue in the navel and have your patient place their hands on the sides of their head so that the hands extend from the sphenoid bone (the temples) along to the area above the ears.

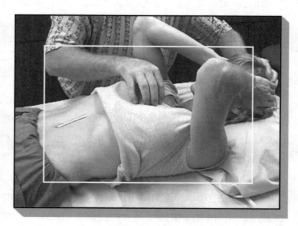

Treating hydration

- *You will then treat the cortices as you did in the cortex treatment.*
- Place your hand on the patient's head at the base of the skull and upper

106

neck. While you hold that position, tap the head and sternum alternating for a full breath cycle.

- Now move your hand up onto the head to the position next to the one you just did. (You are going to systematically cover the whole head.) In the new position, tap out the head and sternum alternating for a full breath.
- This procedure is repeated until you have covered the whole mid-line of the head. It usually takes four positions although small hands on a big head may take five. (You do not need to do the sides of the head as you did with the basic cortices because they are already covered by the patient's hands.)

Sometimes the treatment will need to be repeated or it will not hold well. In those cases, other factors have to be tied into the treatment with advanced techniques.

A common example is the emotional factor. Water is energetically tied to the concept of joy. Often, when a person is rejecting water by not absorbing it, there is a tendency for the person to be rejecting joy in their life. For them 'life is a struggle' and it essentially lacks joy as the common denominator and birthright.

CASE HISTORY:

Sandra was diagnosed with a chronic case of fibromyalgia. All her joints and muscles ached constantly. She had constant headaches and her skin looked old for her age. Hydration showed up very strongly when tested and treated.

For the next few days after her treatment Sandra felt very thirsty and craved water. Interestingly, before the treatment, whenever she was thirsty, Sandra felt like drinking iced tea. Now she only wanted water.

Her joint and muscle pain improved rapidly over the next three weeks and, when I saw her for a follow-up three months later, there was a visible change in her skin texture and looks. She said that she felt like she had been given a face lift all over her body.

CHAPTER

15

Scars and Skin Blockages

IN THIS CHAPTER WE ARE GOING TO LOOK AT AN EXTREMELY IMPORTANT cause of many diseases and health problems. It is also one that is rarely taken into account in health care practices. Scars, when not healed correctly, can cause many blockages in energy flow, circulation, and nerve flow that can affect the body locally or have serious ramifications throughout the body.

A healthy scar is one that is fine, soft, not tender and not raised. Unhealthy scars are usually thicker, often tender, often have redness around them and temperature differences from one side to the other. Unhealthy scars block the flow of energy along the meridian energy pathways and inhibit the function of all the areas supplied by that meridian. Unhealthy scars will also upset the energic hologram of the body by interfering with the general balance of energy throughout the body.

Before the BodyTalk treatment for scars, I used to use an acupuncture treatment whereby I bridged the scar. This means that I placed needles into the scar and in acupuncture points above and below the scar in order to allow the energy to flow through the scar better. This had immediate results and eventually led to the scar partially dissolving and losing its redness and tenderness. Another good scar technique is found in second degree Reiki that has similar results.

By far, BodyTalk has provided the best technique because it is so simple and works quickly. Once the scar has been treated, the release of energy, nerve, and blood flow happens quickly. This gives short-term relief of the symptoms while the scar is healing completely. Eventually, the scar will fade or dissolve into softer tissue and any local coloration or tenderness will go. Not all scars that are creating problems are tender or red. That phenomena is just common in bad cases.

Why Don't Scars Heal Well?

How well a scar heals usually depends upon a few different factors.

• The general health and vitality of the patient at the time. If, at the time of the accident or operation that caused the scar, you are run down, sick, or have poor vitality, then the scar will often heal poorly and give you problems later on.

• The most common cause is emotional stress at the time of the accident or operation. If the accident caused a lot of emotional stress that you did not handle well because of circumstances, then the scar will heal badly. Typically, you may have been injured in a car accident that others were hurt in and this led to a lot of emotional stress at the time. You may have been worried about disfigurement or experienced significant pain that stressed you as well. In other scenarios, you may be having an operation that is very emotional for you. For example, you may have a hysterectomy or body part removed that meant a change in lifestyle or attitudes. This resultant emotional stress will cause poor repair to the scarred area.

Another interesting concept here is that very often BodyTalk practitioners find that the connective tissue associated with the scar will tend to hold the repressed emotions locally around the scar. Often, when treating scars, there will be emotional releases and memories related to the time when the scar occurred.

A common scenario involves the woman who has a successful hysterectomy but then experiences other changes in her body during the months and years after the operation. Typically, she would suffer from depletion in the flow of the yin meridians that flow up the inside the leg, along the front of the trunk, to the head. If the hysterectomy scar blocks the energy flow, the woman will experience deficiency symptoms in the abdomen, chest, and head. There will typically be poor digestion, poor sugar metabolism, tiredness and weakness, shortness of breath, circulatory insufficiency, and poor energy flow to the head causing the facial muscles to start sagging. The list can be endless—all because of that scar.

When the woman complains to the doctor that the problems started after the hysterectomy, she will often be told that it is coincidence because removing the uterus will not give those symptoms. Hundreds of women have experienced transformations in their health after their hysterectomy scar has been treated by BodyTalk.

CASE HISTORY:

Kay had a face-lift and breast implants in a final bid to regain lost youth. The decision to have the operation was very emotional and on reflection she realized that it was also an attempt to save a failing marriage. The whole procedure became a nightmare. The breast implants gave her constant pain and the scars on her breasts and face were clearly visible months later.

In the meantime, internal scars had developed in the breasts causing pain and discomfort. She couldn't bear to be touched on the breasts and they felt hard, abnormal, and were sources of misery contributing further problems to the failing marriage. The face eventually healed and looked satisfactory but she felt constant tension in the facial muscles and she was chronically tired. The BodyTalk scar treatment was performed on the breast scars and the small scars on the scalp caused by the face lift.

Within a week the breasts were softer and less painful. The facial tension totally relaxed and the complexion improved. After five more treatments the breasts were pain free, soft, and the scarring had faded dramatically. Eventually, the internal adhesions in the breasts also dissolved.

Test

- To test to see if a scar is causing problems you need to challenge (poke) the scar while you muscle test. This poke is firm but not

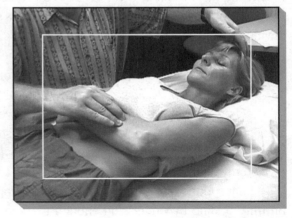

Treating scars and moles

strong enough to cause discomfort.

- You ask, *"Is there a problem with this scar?"* If the answer is *yes* then the scar should be treated.

Treatment

To treat the scar you continue to challenge (poke) the scar repeatedly while you tap out the head and sternum and ask the patient to breathe deeply for two full breath cycles.

Retest

You should then retest the scar to confirm that the correction is successful. Sometimes the scar will need to be treated a few times. On other occasions this simple correction will not be enough. The patient will need advanced BodyTalk treatments to link the scar with other factors. The most common linkage is to the emotions.

It is important that the body is checked thoroughly for scars before any form of energy therapy is given. Some scars are very small and are a problem because they just happen to be on a specific acupuncture point or meridian. This means that, although very small, the scar can cause a significant imbalance in the energy hologram. I have seen scars that are hard to see without a magnifying glass cause problems because they are directly on an acupuncture point.

Sometimes there will be a problem finding the scars. We tend to forget about them, especially if they are small. Other times we won't see them because they are in more intimate areas of the body and covered by clothing.

When you feel you have treated the obvious scars, you can then ask if there are more scars to treat. If the answer is *yes* (weak muscle), then you need to find them by asking a series of questions to locate the scar. For example:

"Is the scar on the trunk?" No (muscle strong)
"Is the scar on the legs?" Yes (muscle weak)
"Is the scar on the left leg?" Yes (muscle weak)
"Is the scar below the knee?" No (muscle strong)
"Is the scar on the front of the thigh?" Yes (muscle weak)

You would then examine the thigh to find the scar and treat it.

I have found tiny scars on fully dressed people. We were then able to confirm my finding by undressing enough to expose the scar exactly where the innate wisdom told me it was!

A little side note here regarding treating scars in places where the patient is reluctant to disrobe. In some countries there are cultural taboos to undressing— even to have their body treated. This makes it a challenge. You can try treating the scar through the clothing. This will often work if the fabric is non-synthetic. If it doesn't work, then I teach the patient how to treat the scar and ask them to have a spouse or family member treat it at home. Otherwise, you just have to accept the fact that some people would rather be sick than expose their body, for whatever reason, and not treat them.

Moles and Blemishes

The scar treatment is also used to treat moles and blemishes. By testing (poking) a mole and testing a muscle, one can determine whether the mole is unhealthy.

The mole or blemish is then treated the same as scars and retested. Very often the patient will notice that the mole will gradually fade back to a healthy color over the next 3-6 weeks. This is very useful for many ugly blemishes and has great significance when one considers the amount of skin cancer present in our society.

There have been many case histories of quite dangerous looking moles fading back into a healthy state quite quickly. In other cases I have seen the mole or blemish drop off after a few days.

CASE HISTORY:

Gerald was 55 years old and had a large, crusty, sunspot on the tip of his nose for two years. It was gradually growing and his doctor wanted to cut it out. Gerald was reluctant to do so because the doctor pointed out that the whole tip of his nose would be removed and require plastic surgery.

He was having a BodyTalk treatment for his back problems when the practitioner automatically treated the sunspot as part of a general treatment to balance the body according to the directions given by his innate wisdom. Ten days later the spot had completely gone leaving nothing at all except slightly shiny skin.

BodyTalk can also be used to treat internal scars and adhesions using advanced linking. Scars and blockages in the form of moles, blemishes, tattoos, and deformities are easily the most overlooked factor in health care. They block energy, nerves, and circulation and will slow up treatment in any health care modality and limit the extent of the results obtained. This is why the treatment of scars is considered an essential treatment protocol in BodyTalk. It needs to be checked during the first treatment for every patient.

CHAPTER

16

Treating the Organs

NOW THAT WE HAVE CORRECTED ALL THE ESSENTIAL BASIC COMPONENTS we can start to balance the rest of the body. In this chapter we will balance the organs.

The BodyTalk System™ has shown clinically that one of the main reasons that organs malfunction and become sick is because they have lost synchronicity with the other parts of the body.

The functioning of an organ is not isolated unto itself. It is part of a symphony of orchestrated and integrated biological functions designed to work in synchronicity to maximize health.

With BodyTalk we will correct any discord in that communication and help to restore normal functioning. Once this is done, the body is often able to heal even the most serious of organ problems.

CASE HISTORY:

Pam had been going to her chiropractor for general spinal problems on and off over a period of a few years. She arrived at the chiropractor's office for her spinal treatment looking very upset. Her story was that she had been having severe stomach pain with diarrhea for over a year. She had been having drug therapy during that time. Recently, she had her stomach examined by a specialist with a scope down her esophagus. He told her that her stomach was severely deteriorated and beyond repair with drugs; she needed to have at least three-quarters of her stomach surgically removed. He was not sure of the outcome or what her lifestyle would be like afterward. The doctor pointed out that it was a serious operation and said she would never be the same again. Her operation was scheduled in three weeks time.

The chiropractor had recently learned BodyTalk and suggested they try it. Pam had two BodyTalk treatments in the same week and by the following week felt much better. A few days before the operation Pam insisted that the specialist reexamine her stomach. After the anesthetic wore off the specialist said her stomach was better. Pam asked, "How much better?" The reply, "totally better!" The specialist had no explanation for the recovery but was skeptical about Pam's story of BodyTalk treatment and suggested that the drugs had suddenly worked.

The basic principle of the organ balancing is that we ask the body which organ it wants to balance as a priority. We then ask (using the yes/no muscle test) which organ we need to link to it. The patient holds one organ and the practitioner holds the other organ while tapping out the head and sternum. It is that simple!

This procedure is repeated until you have made all the combinations of organ links that the innate wisdom requests. For example, in one balancing session you may link the lung to the colon; the liver to the pancreas; and the stomach to the small intestine.

In this chapter you will see photos illustrating the positions you hold your hands on the body to 'contact' the organs. Obviously, in some cases, you are not actually contacting the organs. For example, you cannot touch the lungs or heart through the rib cage. This is where intent and focus comes in as discussed in the earlier chapters. When balancing with energy circuits, the key factor is your intent and focus. If you touch the ribs with the intent of the lungs, the innate wisdom will know what you are doing. If you touch the ribs with the intent to the heart, the heart is the organ that will respond. The exact positioning is not critical. The placing of the hands is simply a focusing tool to help the BodyTalk practitioner and patient know what is being treated.

Let us now go though the balancing (linking) procedure step by step. It is assumed that at this point you have completed all the essential treatments covered so far in this book. This is important because there is no point in trying to

The Organ Positions

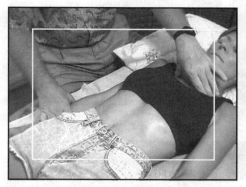

LUNGS

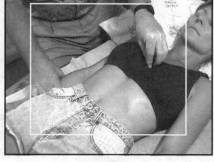

HEART

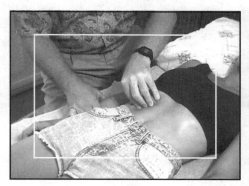

LIVER

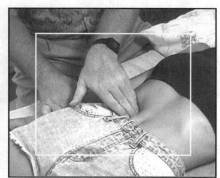

GALL BLADDER

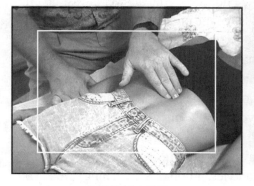

S TOMACH

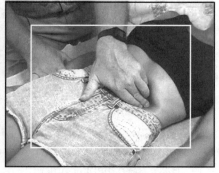

SPLEEN

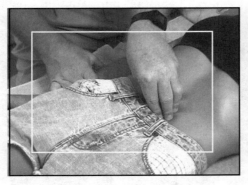

SMALL INTESTINE

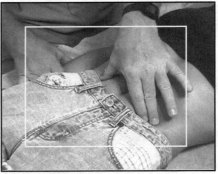

COLON

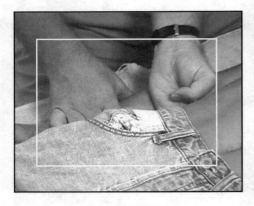

KIDNEYS

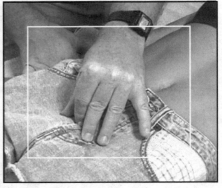

BLADDER

correct an organ if the energy flow through it is being obstructed by a scar or if the cortices of the brain are not balanced to do their function.

- Ask, "Is balancing the organs the priority?" If the answer is *yes*, go on to step two. If the answer is *no*, leave the organs alone and go on to the next section.
- Now systematically place your hands on the organ reflex points illustrated in the photos. Start with the lungs and say, "Is the lung a priority?" If *yes*, go to step 3. If *no*, go to the next organ (heart) and ask if it is the priority. Keep going until you find the priority organ. My suggested order is Lungs, Heart, Liver, Gall Bladder, Stomach, Spleen, Small Intestines, Colon, Bladder, Kidneys.
- Have the patient contact the priority organ (in this case, lung) while you systematically go to each organ and ask if it is the correct link for the

118

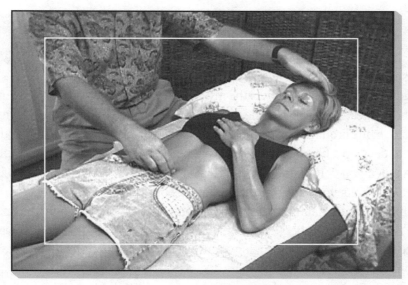

Linking the small intestine to the heart

lung. For example, "Link to heart?" *no*; "Link to liver?" *no*; "Link to stomach?" *yes*. Once you have a *yes*, go to step 4.

- While the patient holds the first organ (in this case—the lung) and the practitioner holds the linked organ (stomach), tap out the head and sternum while the patient takes two full breaths.
- Maintain the contacts and retest to ensure that the problem is corrected. "Is this link now a problem?" *no*.
- You will now ask if there are any further links to the first organ. (In this case, the lungs.) If the answer is *yes*, you then find the next organ to link it to and treat is as before. If the answer is *no*, you start again at step 2 and find the next priority organ that needs to be linked to another organ.

This organ balancing technique can have excellent results in many cases. However, you should remember that this is only part of The BodyTalk System™ of linking. A BodyTalk practitioner will link every aspect of the body. From the organs, he will go on to link the endocrines, and each and every part of the body. In a typical treatment there may be several links in many different combinations.

The following would be a typical series of links:

- Heart to small intestine; heart to adrenals; liver to uterus; pituitary to ovaries; pituitary to pineal; eyes to stomach; diaphragm to bladder;

sacrum to occiput; colon to skin; left limbic brain to right frontal cortex; right limbic brain to adrenals.

If this book inspires you to learn BodyTalk, you may attend the BodyTalk course that will teach you all the linkages. This is very exciting and like playing detective. You gradually unravel the mystery of why that person was ill by utilizing the greatest intelligence in the universe—the innate wisdom of the bodymind. The technique is quite simple. There are occasionally complex links and you will need to develop a broad knowledge of all the links that are possible. You cannot ask a link if you don't know about it. The more you know, the greater the smorgasbord of links you can offer the innate wisdom as a choice.

This is a fascinating concept. I have found that if you have only the knowledge contained in this book, good results will occur. The body will find a way to utilize the links you know, bringing about a series of energy shifts that will correct the physiology of the body.

If you only know eight organs, the body will ask for a series of links to utilize that knowledge. If you also know seven endocrines, then the body now has a total of fifteen components it can combine in different links. That is a sudden huge jump in possible combinations. A BodyTalk practitioner knows hundreds of links. Imagine the number of combinations.

My experience has been that the more links you know the less links the body makes to correct a condition. For example, if the body needs to correct the function of your thyroid gland and you can only offer it the organs to play with, then it will need to do some pretty fancy linking over a few treatments to indirectly influence and correct the thyroid.

If, however, the endocrines are available as links, it may only need to link the pituitary to the thyroid and the thyroid to the liver to correct the problem in one visit.

The simple techniques taught in this book are safe and will help a lot of problems very well. Please remember, however, that this book is only scratching the surface of BodyTalk. For comprehensive results, you will need to visit a BodyTalk practitioner or, if you wish to become a BodyTalk practitioner, you will need to enroll in one of our workshops.

CASE HISTORY:

Jim was having a lot of digestive problems. He always felt tired, headachy, and bloated after eating and had a lot of flatulence. He felt that he never digested his food well and noticed undigested food in his stools.

The BodyTalk treatment corrected the essential basics and then linked: liver to small intestine; liver to pancreas; gall bladder to small intestine; stomach to colon.

Within a week Jim's digestion was back to normal. His energy increased dramatically over the following few weeks and the headaches were gone.

Blood Chemistry

THE TREATMENTS TAUGHT IN THIS CHAPTER ARE REALLY WHAT ESTAB-
lished BodyTalk as a potential major treatment modality. When I talk of body
chemistry, I am referring to many factors including viruses, infections, parasites,
allergies, food intolerances, toxic chemicals, etc. and all the unwanted elements
in our system. The treatment described later in this chapter will enable you to
help remedy most of these factors. It will not treat everything because what I am
covering in this book is a simplified version. This will usually solve about 60% of
the virus cases for example. For the tough cases, you will need to know the rest
of The BodyTalk System™. In the full treatment protocol, as taught in my BodyTalk
Modules 1 and 2, there are many other links that give the body far greater
options with regard to treatment.

For example, many food intolerances, allergies, or chronic viruses are
strongly linked to emotional factors. In these cases, the body chemistry treatment then has to be linked to the emotional treatment to clear the specific emotional event in the patient's life that started the problem.

However, the treatment in this chapter is safe, easy, and will help the majority of cases spectacularly. Often, only one treatment is necessary and results
are seen within hours. If a family member comes down with an infection, acute
virus, or allergy, it means that you can try the BodyTalk treatment first and look

for fast results. If the results aren't there, you can visit your professional BodyTalk practitioner who knows the whole system or, if one is not available, go to your doctor for conventional medication.

Viruses

The treatment of viruses has long been a problem for the medical profession, and to this day the treatment of viruses basically involves trying to get the body healthy enough to treat the virus itself. There are no effective anti-viral treatments that will directly kill a virus in the same way antibodies can kill bacteria.

With The BodyTalk System™ we address the problem directly by simply highlighting the presence of the virus to the body and asking it to treat that virus by launching an immune attack on the virus. Before doing this we will have prepared and balanced the body with the essential basic treatments covered earlier and linked the required organs.

In chronic conditions, one of the main problems is that the virus stays in the system for years creating havoc and causing many symptoms of chronic fatigue syndrome, fibromyalgia, and numerous other illnesses. In these cases the body's defense system is either unable to recognize the presence of the virus, or reluctant to take on the virus because the system is too run down or weak to tackle the virus. This occurs when the lines of communication are not functioning correctly and the synchronicity of the organs is compromised.

We all know that a general would be reluctant to fight a war if his troops were not trained to synchronize their movements and the communication systems were not working. The BodyTalk System™ corrects the communication breakdown by balancing and linking the system to create a readiness for the body to take on the job.

The treatment of bacteria has also become a problem for general health care professionals because, while antibiotics may serve us well initially, nature fights back. We now find ourselves in the situation where bacteria are becoming resistant to normal antibiotics. Over the years, the pharmacological industry has produced stronger antibiotics which, unfortunately, have many side effects because they kill the healthy bacteria while killing the infection. This is also compounded by the emergence of 'super' bacteria that are resistant to many antibiotics and, in some cases, all known antibiotics.

A major problem here is that it is very difficult to produce the specific antibody necessary to kill a specific bacterium. The antibodies tend to have a broad spectrum effect killing everything in their path.

In The BodyTalk System™ we pinpoint the infection and ask the body to specifically treat that infection. The immune response then responds by producing a specific antibody that will *target that infection only*. The fact that this can occur is great news for all of us because it means that we can treat infections without the hazardous side effects of killing off all our healthy bacteria every time we have a treatment. For most people the taking of a course of antibiotics weakens their whole immune system, causes their candidia population to grow unchecked, and takes weeks or months to reestablish a healthy intestinal flora.

Although The BodyTalk System™ may not kill off all bacteria as fast as is necessary in some acute cases, the fact that it will do it in most cases has to be one of the great news flashes in health care for the 21st century!

CASE HISTORY:

Jenny was diagnosed with fibromyalgia at age 26. By the time she came to me, at 35, Jenny was in constant pain, extremely fatigued, headaches daily, and every part of her body felt sore and painful to touch. Using the BodyTalk protocol I established that several organs were not in healthy communication and had to link: liver to pancreas, kidneys to colon, and stomach to colon. I then asked her body if there was any infections or viruses present and the answer was yes. Her innate wisdom detected three viruses and two infections, all chronic. After the treatment was given, Jenny noticed a slight increase in body temperature and within three hours her temperature had risen to 103° F. For the next three days she had a mild temperature and stayed in bed because she felt extra tired from all the healing that was going on.

One week later I saw her again and she felt significantly improved. She was less tired, no headaches, and in less pain. Her body indicated that one virus was still present and that was treated using the treatment in this chapter. Her innate wisdom said to give another treatment in one month. One month later Jenny arrived beaming and gave me a huge hug. No symptoms were left! I just gave her a general balancing to ensure that everything would be maintained and her health would remain robust.

CASE HISTORY:

Paul was 10 years old and had come to me for a second visit regarding a dyslexia problem he had. His mother mentioned that there was a infection going around his school and Paul had caught it. His throat was very sore, he had a cough producing greenish phlegm and he was very tired. His mother had booked him in with their doctor for later that day but asked if I could do anything since she didn't want to give Paul more antibiotics. Apparently Paul had received two previous courses in the past two months.

The BodyTalk treatment indicated that he had both an infection and a virus—both acute. I treated him with BodyTalk as described in this book. His mother cancelled the doctor's appointment. The next day she phone me to say that Paul woke up feeling well and went to school.

Parasites

Parasites are another major problem in health care. Evidence is now pointing to parasites as being far more prevalent than most people realize. The most common parasites are those found in the intestines from food intake. They cause diarrhea, nausea and vomiting if in an acute phase. Sometimes the symptoms settle down and they stay in the intestines creating digestive and intestinal irritations. When your doctor tests your stools for parasites, these are what will show in that test. There are drugs to kill the parasites but they are very powerful and many patients feel the treatment is as bad as the complaint! They can also leave you feeling ill and run down for months since the drugs are quite toxic.

The BodyTalk treatment will kill most of these parasites within a day or two; often occurring within a few hours. Out of the hundreds of intestinal parasite treatments I have given, so far there has only been one case that still required the drugs. (Some of the big parasites from South America are pretty tough.)

CASE HISTORY:

Terry went to the British Virgin Islands a few weeks after a major hurricane hit. She was there helping in restorations. On her previous trips she had drunk the local water out of the tap because it was excellent. Out of habit she did it again even though everyone is warned not to drink the water untreated after a hurricane as the water tables and sewerage tables have a habit of meeting and mixing.

Terry came into my office with two buckets—one for each end. She was extremely ill. Her innate wisdom told me that she had seven different types of parasites in her body. Four of them in her intestines. She also had a bowel infection.

When I saw her the next day the severe diarrhea and vomiting had stopped but she was still quite ill. Further tests indicated that one of the parasites was still there. I treated her again and had to do further more complex links to her endocrines and lymphatic system. Two days later she was well. No drugs were taken.

That parasites exist in the intestines is common knowledge and they are treated one way or the other by many health care practitioners. One form of parasites that many do not take into account are micro-parasites that can get through the intestinal walls, body orifices, and skin. They lodge themselves in the organs, endocrine glands, lymphatic vessels, and anywhere they can hide and colonize. They do not produce major symptoms of their own and tend to live, undetected, in an area for years. The main danger with these parasites is in the way they affect the function of their host. Chronic parasites in an organ will damage it eventually. When they are in the endocrine glands they cause malfunctioning of that gland.

These parasites cannot be detected through normal laboratory tests. The stool test only (sometimes) detects parasites located in the intestines. I spoke to a pathologist patient and asked if he had seen micro-parasites in endocrine glands and his answer was yes. "How do you detect them?" I asked. His answer was simple, "In autopsies!"

CASE HISTORY:

Rusty had a long history of fatigue, sugar cravings, and stress management problems. He also had chronic backache around his kidney area that was worse when he was tired. He had been having extensive therapy from conventional and alternative health care practitioners. As part of the BodyTalk treatment I routinely asked if there were parasites and the answer was yes. Then, I asked the body for their specific location. (A technique taught in our BodyTalk workshops.) The answer was that he had micro-parasites in the adrenal glands. (Theses glands are located over the kidneys and accounted for his backache when he was tired.)

Treatment of the parasites involved the body chemistry treatment as described later in this chapter and I also had to link his adrenals to his liver and pancreas to stabilize his blood sugar. I also linked his adrenals to the pituitary gland to correct the way his body handled stress. The one treatment cleared his health problems over the next two weeks.

Allergies

It is difficult to find a way to treat allergies that gives permanent results. The simple blood chemistry treatment you are about to learn will help simple cases very effectively. A typical seasonal reaction to oak tree pollen, for example, will usually respond within an hour and last for the season. In a fairly healthy person with mild allergies this treatment is magic. In tough cases of life long multiple severe allergies you will find this treatment only gives temporary relief except for the occasional 'miracle'. When the allergies are serious, the complete BodyTalk protocol has to be used by a fully trained BodyTalk practitioner.

The same applies for food allergies and environmental toxins such as mercury poisoning. Simple cases respond well to the techniques taught in this book. Tough cases will respond very well to BodyTalk but require the whole protocol to give permanent results.

CASE HISTORY:

Alan came in for treatment to his back, strained by gardening. He was also choked up in the nose and throat with red eyes and looked miserable. He explained that he had mowed and gardened under his pine trees the day before and was reacting to the pollen as he did every year at that time. He did not want to take drugs because he reacted to them and they left him feeling nonfunctional.

He was not aware that BodyTalk treated allergies and was happy about the prospect of having his allergies fixed at the same time as his back. I saw him a week later for a follow-up and his back was improving, but the allergies had gone the day after I treated him. He had spent more time in the garden with no ill effects.

The Blood Chemistry Treatment

- At this point you will have performed all the techniques covered in this book on the patient. Those techniques are very important because they prepare the patient so that the bodymind is able to respond appropriately to any subsequent form of treatment.
- You now ask "Is there a problem with blood chemistry?" If the answer is *yes*, go on to the next step. (If the answer is *no,* it means that even if there is a problem, the body is not prepared to treat it at the moment. It may be that the body wants a few hours or days to correct itself more

128

from the earlier treatments. It may also simply mean that there are no problems in this area. (Healthy people do actually exist!)

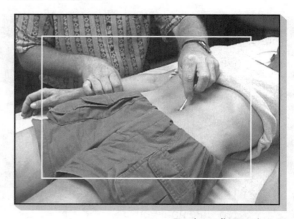

Testing saliva on tissue

- Take a Q-tip or small piece of tissue and rub it on the patient's gums to get a sample of saliva and traces of blood. This will provide you with the point of reference for the body. The Q-tip is placed on a high energy center of the body so that the innate wisdom can 'read' it. I suggest that the best place is in the navel (belly button). If that is hard to access because of clothing, the left ear or the sternum can be used. This saliva-soaked Q-tip now becomes the focus of information with which the innate wisdom gathers knowledge of what is going on specifically within the body.

- Ask (using your muscle test) what the priority problem is. For example, "Is there a virus? If *yes,* go to step three to treat the virus. If *no*, ask the next question. "Is there an infection?" If *yes*, treat the infection. If *no* ask further until you find what the body wants to treat. Sample questions: "Is there a parasite?" "Is there an allergy?" "Is there a toxin?"

- Make sure you and the patient are aware of what you are treating (for example, virus) and have the patient place their hands on either side of their head. The hands will cover the temples to the upper half of their ears. This connects the limbic part of the brain to the treatment that is vital for results. (The reason for this is not covered in this book—just be happy with the clinical results!)

- While the patient keeps their hands on the sides of their heads you will then treat the cortices as you did in the cortex treatment. That is:
  1) Place your hand on the patient's head at the base of the skull and upper neck. While you hold that position, tap the head and sternum, alternating for a full breath cycle.
  2) Now move your hand up onto the head to the position next to the one

129

you just did. (You are going to systematically cover the whole head.) In the new position, tap out the head and sternum alternating for a full breath.

3) This procedure is repeated until you have covered the

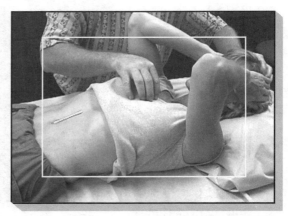

Treating saliva to cortices

whole mid-line of the head. It usually takes four positions although small hands on a big head may take five. (You do not need to do the sides of the head as you did with the basic cortices since they are already covered by the patient's hands.)

Retest

Now retest for the condition you treated (for example, virus) by asking, "Is there a virus?" If the answer is *no*, move on to the next question (infection, parasites, etc.).

Sometimes the answer will be *yes* there is a virus after you have treated one. This is because you have to treat a second virus specifically. You can ask "Is this a second virus? If the answer is *yes,* then you have to do the whole treatment again for the second virus. On other occasions you will have treated several viruses in the one treatment. This can sometimes be confusing and in the workshop we teach a protocol to sort this all out. In fact we can ask exactly how many viruses, infections, etc. exist and where they are. This is interesting sometimes, although when it comes down to results, all that really matters is that you do the treatment as described and the patient gets better.

One important part of the treatment to remember is that when you treat a virus the body goes through a healing immune response. This means that in many cases the temperature of the body will go up for a few hours or even a few days. This is a natural part of the healing process. In acute viruses, the patient will not really notice a difference because they will already have a temperature. In chronic viruses, however, the patient may be quite surprised by the sudden increase in temperature as the body is healing. It is best to warn them that this could happen so they don't panic.

Another consideration is when the patient's blood has been monitored for viruses. They may have a pathology report that indicates they have the Epstein-Barr virus in their system. You need to realize that these pathology tests are measuring the existence of antibodies or antigens in the system. Pathology tests usually do not measure the actual virus because most viruses cannot be measured directly.

When you treat a chronic virus with BodyTalk and the patient has blood tests a week later, they may be told that their virus is much worse because their 'count' has gone up sharply. However, when the doctor sees a very healthy patient in front of him, he will realize that the test needs to be interpreted differently. The doctor should then realize that the high count is an indication that the body has gone through an immune response and has increased the antibodies dramatically to kill off the virus. In this case, the high count is a good sign.

The treatment I have just covered is very exciting. It promises hope for the millions suffering from the effects of chronic and acute viruses, infections, parasites, and the whole spectrum of chemical toxins and allergic reactions. As mentioned at the beginning of the chapter, there are stubborn cases that require more knowledge of BodyTalk for the desired result. I am sure there will be some cases that do not respond and require the use of drug therapy.

In the meantime, you can safely try the treatment out on your friends and family and change their lives. Remember, if the condition is serious and you are not sufficiently trained, do not wait long to seek more professional help.

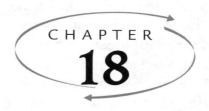

CHAPTER

18

Treating the Chakras

THE FOLLOWING FEW PAGES ARE PRIMARILY EXTRACTED FROM *REIKI: THE Science, Metaphysics, and Philosophy*, the book I co-authored with my wife Esther. Many systems of healing are excellent at treating and balancing the Chakras. Reiki is one such system that obtains excellent results. I have modified sections to make it applicable to BodyTalk.

In this chapter I will be explaining the importance of the Chakras and their function. At the end of the chapter I will teach you how to use the BodyTalk system to effectively balance the chakras within the BodyTalk protocol.

Numerous books have been written on the subject of the chakras—the body's "generator system." It is impossible to do the subject justice in one chapter. In order to understand the magnitude of BodyTalk's potential as a facilitator for personal/spiritual growth, a minimal understanding of these energy centers is helpful.

Our physical body comprises various levels of vibratory rates of energy. Within our gross (i.e. tangible) physical body there exist numerous energy centers of yet higher frequencies than those previously acknowledged by science. These centers were long ago acknowledged by mystics in various parts of the world. The term chakra comes from the Sanskrit meaning "circle of movement." It is variously translated as "vortex of spinning energy" or "wheel."

There are purportedly over three hundred of these energy centers in the body. This chapter will focus on the seven major chakras.

After conception, the earliest stages of embryological development focus on the cerebrospinal system. It is through the cerebrospinal system that the body receives its life force. The seven major chakras are high frequency psychic/energy centers situated in close proximity to the cerebrospinal system. These energy centers may be likened to the energy generators of the developing organism.

As *centers of transformation* the chakras step down subtle energies and transform them into nerve, cellular and hormonal energy within the physical body. The conduits, or subtle "pathways" which facilitate this interchange between psychological and physical energy, are called nadis.

Various scientific studies have finally given credibility to the existence of the chakras. As a result, science is now beginning to acknowledge what the mystics have long been teaching regarding their importance in relation to the physiological level. Dysfunction at the level of the chakras and nadis is directly reflected in pathological disorders within the nervous system and endocrine system that, in turn, will affect the whole bodymind. The chakras are closely linked to higher consciousness and, therefore, to our innate wisdom. Correctly functioning chakras are vital for the innate wisdom to do its job in synchronizing the entire bodymind system.

The physical, mental and spiritual aspects of the body work together and are interconnected. It is, therefore, important to remember that any disorder at the physiological level will always be, to some extent, reflected at the subtler levels and visa versa. The following information is a brief summary of the dynamics of the chakras from an emotional, mental, physiological, and spiritual standpoint.

The seven major chakras have many concordances. This chapter addresses only those relevant to our purpose. The concordance of primary importance is that of the endocrine glands. The endocrine system affects the supply of hormonal secretions into the blood stream. These secretions determine growth rate, sexual development, and numerous physiological activities.

The chakras also have corresponding organs, qualities, emotions, colors, and elements. Information regarding the chakras varies but we must realize that there are levels within levels when one addresses this subject. Herein we only skim the surface of an immense and highly refined system.

Base Chakra

The first chakra is situated at the area of the genitalia (base of the spine) and is referred to as the base chakra in English. This chakra is associated with the kidneys and the adrenal glands. The associated element is earth. The emotion or "quality" associated with this chakra is the emotion of fear.

At this stage it is important to understand that *the chakras are seats of consciousness through which we express ourselves.* Perhaps we should say, ideally, we express ourselves through them, but in most cases we consciously—or unconsciously—limit expression to but a couple of these centers.

During the first seven years of development, ideally, we express ourselves through this first seat of consciousness. We are mainly interested in being fed, nurtured, having our diapers changed and basically *surviving.* For this reason the base chakra is also often referred to as the survival chakra.

As adults, if we continue to express ourselves healthily through this seat of consciousness, we are grounded people (hence the earth element association). We are highly motivated because the emotion of fear activates the "flight or fight" response when necessary and gives us our get-up-and-go. We have a good sense of our place in relation to the material world and feel secure within it.

Limited expression through the base chakra is often reflected in insecurity when relating to the material world. This may result in violent or avaricious behavior. The person will feel generally "ungrounded" and at odds with his/her environment or simply detached from it. The person with a weak base chakra will always have difficulty in manifesting and/or managing money, etc. They will often be referred to a 'space cadets' and have difficulty in settling into a stable lifestyle.

Sexual Chakra

From approximately the seventh year of life until the age of about fourteen, we begin to discover our sensual/sexual body. A new awareness of our physical body and our individuality develops. Along with it evolves our imagination and creativity.

This chakra is linked to the yin aspect of the kidneys, the ovaries in women, and the testes and prostate in men. It is related to the element of water (essence of life) and has to do with the fluid flows of the body: blood, urine, lymph, etc.

A person who is well centered in this chakra is someone with healthy body awareness and high self-love/esteem. The person will express his/her individuality living creatively. He/she will have a healthy regard and relationship with his or her sexuality and its expression and as a result be deeply in touch with joy.

Unfortunately few of us express ourselves healthily through this seat of consciousness. Early on, as we enter the period associated with the development of expression through the sexual chakra, many of us are told "you are big now and shouldn't walk around without clothes on" (i.e. masks are necessary and there is reason to hide this part of you), "don't touch yourself," etc. Young women learn about "the curse" and all kinds of horrendous trials and tribulations of being female. Young men are rarely taught enough to assuage fears of the mysteries of the female.

Incest, child-beating, and touch-starvation are sad facts in many people's lives. If we receive negative programming about our physical/sensual body, we learn quickly to close down sensitivity to it. We cease expressing ourselves through this chakra because it is "unacceptable" to society and painful to us. If we do so, we may suffer from an inability to experience sexual pleasure or to express ourselves sensually and creatively. Invariably feelings of inadequacy at this level are reflected in possessive, jealous personalities.

Ovarian cysts/tumors, breast problems (all links to the reproductive system), sterility, impotency, premenstrual syndrome, obsessive/compulsive sexual behavior, etc., may be signs that, on some level, we have chosen to cease healthy expression through the sexual chakra.

Lack of self-expression at this level is the basis for the majority of our disease processes in life. If we reject our physical body, we reject self. Self-rejection depletes the immune system. Rejection of our sensuality/sexuality causes depression of our life-force energy. We stay out of touch with our innate capacity for joy, or limit it dramatically.

Solar Plexus Chakra

By the time we are about fourteen years of age, we reach the stage where we begin to develop our own sense of personal power (in the positive sense of the word) and the ability to manifest our dreams. Because most of us struggled uncomfortably with the first two chakras, by the time we are at this stage our sense of personal power is often distorted, limited or non-existent.

The solar plexus chakra is associated with the stomach (digestion), spleen

136

(transformation and purification of blood), pancreas (secretes digestive juice, pancreatin, and insulin), liver (produces bile and converts carbohydrates into energy/glucogens), and the gall bladder (stores bile). These are our organs of digestion and assimilation, not just of food, but of emotions.

In a healthy organism, when the body has finished the process of digesting and assimilating food, it continues with an organic process of emotional synthesis. We are under the misconception that the rumbling of the tummy means we need food. Tummy rumbles are a sign of peristalsis (muscular contractions of the alimentary and intestinal canals) that affects expulsion of waste. Peristalsis often denotes synthesis at the emotional level.

We have all had times when we are upset and either gorge or starve ourselves as a coping mechanism. What we are actually doing is halting the body's natural emotional synthesizing process. We get "the runs" in sympathy with the bottom falling out of our lives, or we suffer from constipation, reflecting our insecurity and need to cling to the old and familiar, however uncomfortable that may be.

The third chakra is related to the emotion of anger. Since few of us are in touch with our own personal power, anger is usually in excess (whether expressed outwardly, stifled or even projected onto a "nagging" partner). By the time we reach the solar plexus chakra most of us are candidates for stomach ulcers, liver cancer, hypoglycemia, digestive problems, or a combination thereof.

If we are healthily centered and expressing ourselves through this chakra, we have a high self-esteem and natural ability to manifest—and enjoy—abundance on all levels. The solar plexus chakra is linked to the liver, which, in metaphysics, is the seat of the soul. Here we begin to develop a healthy relationship with self, which is reflected in our interaction with our environment.

Those of us who struggle at the level of the third chakra may have distorted, overblown egos to mask our inner insecurities about our role in relationship to the outer world. Another method for dealing with our inability to express through this seat of consciousness is to introvert. We keep everything bottled up like a time bomb and probably live in a hostile environment that is merely mirroring the turmoil of our own psyche.

The element associated with the solar plexus chakra is fire. Fire is the element of transformation. Leave it unattended and it can become harmful and burn out of control (excess/violent) or simply go out (deficient/unmotivated).

Heart Chakra

As the quality of the heart chakra is self-love, it is the chakra through which many of us have a great deal of trouble expressing ourselves.

The heart chakra is considered the seat of balance in the body. It is associated not only with the heart, but also the lungs and thymus (immune system). The associated element is air.

The heart chakra anchors the life force—our breathing. It is our breathing that effects movement of the rib cage and consequent massaging of our vital organs beneath it. This massaging action directly affects how well, or how poorly, our digestion and assimilation processes work.

So, what do we do? When we are upset we have great ways of avoiding synthesizing our emotions. We chain smoke, which is a wonderful way to diminish the efficacy of the lungs and an effective way of stifling emotions. Another method is to hold our breath or breathe shallowly. We are all pretty expert in the art of how *not* to breathe. In fact, considering that it is this very process that keeps us alive, it is amazing how many of us have never learned to do it properly. My earlier chapter on breath and its relevance in BodyTalk will also show how important it is to have the heart chakra synchronized with the rest of the body as well as the other chakras.

Those of us in the above category are classic candidates for lung cancer, pneumonia (water/tears in the lungs), heart disease, etc.

In the military, soldiers are trained in "correct" posture: head up, shoulders back; an excellent way of armoring the heart center to avoid having to feel emotions when entering the battlefield. Unfortunately many of us were trained this way at home and in school. Breast implants are another good way of armoring the heart center and very effective in blocking energy flow in the body. Most of us are actually experts in avoiding expression through this center.

The physiological effect, on the thymus, of true laughter and smiling is strength. Just being in touch with joy will strengthen the immune system. The connection between a healthy immune system and self-love is undeniable. When we look at the number of immune system disorders in our society today, it is indicative of the underdeveloped heart chakra most of us have.

You know what it feels like to fall in love. Suddenly everything seems to go right, you feel better about yourself and can express yourself to this person like you never have to anyone else. Even your health problems seem to diminish! When we are with that someone we deem special we feel more creative, more intelligent, more beautiful.

We spend a lot of time dreaming of falling in love and trying to find someone to fall in love with. We may be in love with that person's creative talent, intellect, ability to interact, or beauty. Whatever draws us to another person (consciously or unconsciously) is usually an aspect of ourselves we see reflected in that person. When we are with him or her, our heart chakra expands, and becomes more dynamic. As a result, we experience the specialness within ourselves.

At first the feelings are of bliss and joy because we are seeing ourselves through the beloved's eyes and self-love is possible. Sadly, most of us are so used to giving away our power (under-functioning solar plexus chakra) that we continue to project what is special about us onto our beloved. We refuse to own it and fail to appreciate the reflection our beloved is offering us of our own specialness. As a result we become disillusioned with him/her and "fall" out of love.

The reason our ability to love is conditional is because we are requiring the other person to make us special. How can we possibly think we are being honest when we say "I love you" to someone if we do not even know how to love ourselves? What we are really saying is "I love you...because you *make me feel* a certain way": "You are in total control of my emotions." We are giving away our power and putting tremendous pressure on our partners to be custodians of our emotional stability, thereby setting ourselves up for disappointment (a misnomer frequently used instead of the word anger).

Those of us who have decided to be "selfless" and work and slave to make our family happy or save the world could be misguided. Probably, the best thing we can do for the world is to begin by expressing ourselves through our heart chakra, that is, loving self. If we, as the microcosm, have internal battles with self going on, how can we possibly expect the macrocosm to reflect peace and unity? We are hypocritical if we profess to be devoting our lives to "fixing" the world if we aren't also working to heal our relationship with ourselves.

Ideally, if we are healthily expressing through the heart chakra and have a good relationship with self, then the possibility that the rest of our chakras are dynamic and healthy is increased. The heart is considered the seat of balance in the body, making self-love the key to a healthy chakra system.

If you love yourself and then fall in love with someone else, the chances of a healthy enduring relationship are high. The new expansion to your heart chakra will allow the energy to flow more dynamically out to the other chakras. We "fall in love" and take the energy down to our solar plexus chakra and synthesize it.

Ideally, we then take it down to our sexual chakra and express ourselves sensually/sexually to our beloved. We then allow the energy to flow to our base chakra and seek to put down roots (earth element) together, marry, have babies, a white picket fence, etc.

Our inner attitudes about self are often reflected in the kinds of people we draw into our lives. We have but to look around us to see what we really want. It is reflected in what we already have. If we shake our heads and say, "No way, this is the furthest thing from what I want," be sure that some part of you believes this is what you deserve and need right now. If we look at our reality from this perspective, it adds incentive to develop a loving relationship with self. In The BodyTalk System™ we often need to combine the chakra treatment with the emotional treatments to strengthen the heart energy system and irradiate any negative belief systems imprinted in our psyche at a very young age.

Throat Chakra

The throat chakra is associated with the thyroid gland (secretes thyroxin which regulates metabolic rate thus influencing growth and development); the parathyroid gland (produces hormones regulating metabolism of calcium and phosphorous), and the hypothalamus (regulates body temperature). The hypothalmus is sometimes associated with the brow chakra.

On a physiological level, an imbalance in self-expression through the throat chakra will be reflected in under-functioning of the aforementioned organs and glands. This may result in hypothyroidism, characterized by a sluggish metabolism and weight problems. The contrary may be the case, which is hyperthyroidism.

Imbalance at this level may show up in an inability to express oneself verbally or to communicate well. If we have difficulty bringing our deep inner-knowing, thoughts and emotions together in verbal expression, it may be a sign that we need to give more focus to this chakra.

Poets, orators, and singers make up some of the realm of creative people centered in this chakra. Ether is the element associated with this chakra, which amalgamates the first four chakras to become sound.

A person truly centered in this chakra will not voice intellectually or emotionally programmed belief systems. Rather, they are more likely to speak from a place of knowing and deep inner truth.

Brow Chakra

It is from the sixth chakras that we project our inner dreams outward and manifest them on the physical level. Here is our seat of intuition, insight, and creativity. Here we begin to ask questions of the Spirit, questioning our existence and interrelationship with the universe.

This chakra is associated with the pituitary gland, which functions rather like the orchestral conductor of all the other glands. Directly or indirectly, this gland regulates the majority of basic bodily functions.

If we are "closed minded" and only focus outwardly upon the material aspects of our life, we avoid self-expression through this chakra. We may suffer from eye problems (not wishing to see the truth), or severe headaches. We will only believe in that which we experience with our five senses and probably even have diminished experience through those, meaning that our lower chakras will probably be underdeveloped.

Crown Chakra

In the crown chakra, we experience the meeting of heaven and earth. It is here that your Higher Self or inner spark (whatever term you may use that has meaning for you) interacts with the outer world. If you are balanced and centered in this chakra, one is reflected within the other. The presence of the Divine and the Divine within Self are experienced. The innate wisdom is truly freed to perform its tasks in peak efficiency.

TREATMENT OF THE CHAKRAS

The treatment with BodyTalk is very simple. It follows the same pattern as with organs.

- We have to touch the focus point of each of the chakras (see photos) starting from the base chakra and ask, "Is there a problem with this chakra?" If the answer is *yes*, go to step 2. If the answer is *no*, ask the next chakra.
- Have the patient touch that chakra and look for the chakra to which it has a link. For example, the sexual (2) chakra may have indicated first. The patient places her hands over the chakra while you ask for the link. Is it 3? (solar plexus) If the answer is *yes*, go to step 3. If the answer is *no*, ask for the next link.

- The patient holds one chakra and the practitioner holds the other while tapping out the head and sternum as the patient takes two full deep breaths.
- Check that link has been corrected by asking the link again.
- Ask if there are any further links to that chakra (in this case chakra (2), the sexual chakra.) If the answer is *yes*, find the new link to be treated as in step 3. If the answer is *no*, move on to the next chakra, and so on until you have corrected all the links the innate wisdom requires.

There are few case histories with the chakra treatment because they are usually indirect in influencing tangible results. Balancing the chakras will affect the whole system and the general effectiveness of the entire BodyTalk treatment.

Many patients will, however, report a sudden increase in their feelings of wellbeing. They will feel more centered and relaxed after the treatment. One interesting side effect of the chakra treatment is success in treating many forms of insomnia, especially in children.

CASE HISTORY:

Janice was 8 years old and had a lot of hyperactive symptoms. One of the worst symptoms was her inability to get to sleep at night without medication. The child psychologist treating her taught her mother how to balance the chakras. For three nights in a row the mother found that Janice's heart and crown chakra needed balancing. Each night she fell asleep quickly after the treatment. For the next few months the mother found that she needed to rebalance the chakras about once a week until Janice fell into good sleeping patterns most nights.

I do not normally like BodyTalk treatments to be given as an isolated treatment. However, in the case of the chakra treatment, I have found it to be quite effective to use as a stand-alone treatment for cases like insomnia and to help someone feel more centered and calm the system. More difficult cases will obviously need the full BodyTalk treatment approach.

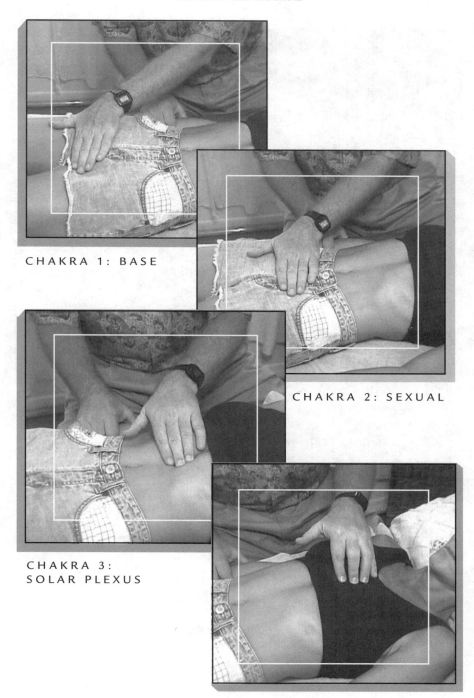

CHAKRA 1: BASE

CHAKRA 2: SEXUAL

CHAKRA 3:
SOLAR PLEXUS

CHAKRA 4: HEART

143

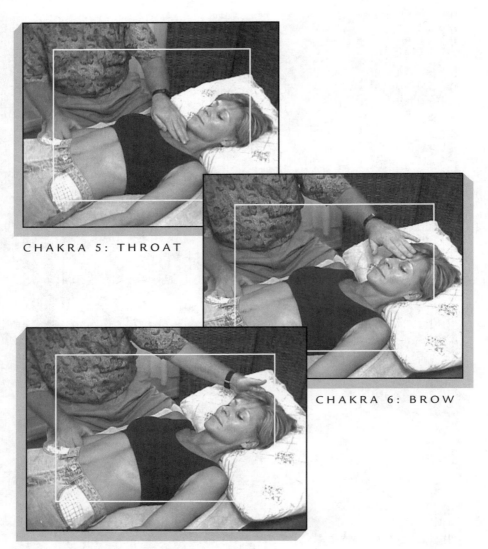

CHAKRA 5: THROAT

CHAKRA 6: BROW

CHAKRA 7: CROWN

Treatment Summary

IN THE PRECEDING CHAPTERS YOU HAVE BEEN SHOWN SEVERAL TREAT-
ments that can be used safely to help your family, friends, or, in the case of
health care practitioners, your patients. I am now going to summarize those
treatments so that you can use these pages as a guide when treating someone
until you have learned everything by heart.

I want to point out that the best thing to do is to go through the whole
system with the people close to you. A few of the essential treatments only need
to be done a few times and they are fixed. For example, you should treat all the
scars on your children until they no longer indicate as needing further treatment.
In this way, if you are treating a child for a bout of influenza, you won't need to
redo the scar treatment as part of the treatment for an acute flu. This can also be
true for vivaxis.

As a general rule, you should always work through the entire system you
have learned whenever you are treating for any condition. The exceptions being
the scars and vivaxis as mentioned in the previous paragraph. For example, a flu
virus will not respond well if you haven't already balanced the lungs to the other
organs if that is necessary. Food allergies will not respond well if you have not
balanced the liver and pancreas appropriately.

Remember, with BodyTalk there are no formulas. Every person, even if they have the same symptoms, will usually need different linkages for their particular system. You must always follow what the innate wisdom of the body is telling you; so that your results are always going to be as fast and complete as possible.

Basic BodyTalk Procedures

The SB Joint

To Test for SB Problems:

- Ask the patient to take a deep breath right in and ask, "Is there a problem with the SB?" If the patient tests *yes* (weak), then they have a problem with their SB locked down. (A scenario like the blow to the head.)
- Then ask the patient to breathe all the way out—right out, as far as possible. Ask, "Is there a problem with SB?" If the patient tests *yes* (weak), then they have a problem with the SB locked up. (The typical startled child reflex.)

To Treat SB Problems:

- Have the patient place their index finger inside their mouth so that they are touching the hard palate (roof of the mouth) almost as far back as the start of the soft palate.
- Place your finger on the pituitary spot, which is the bridge of

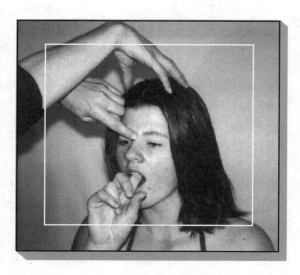

Treatment of the S.B. Joint

the nose where the nose joins the forehead.

- With both these contacts being held, use your spare hand to tap the head and sternum while the patient is asked to take two full deep breaths.

Vivaxis

Testing for Vivaxis

The patient stands with one arm extended at right angles to the body, horizontal to the ground. The practitioner tests the arm by saying, "Is there a problem with vivaxis?" If the test is *no* (a strong arm), then the patient rotates to another point of the compass. Usually I have them rotate about 45° at a time. Each location is tested until there is a *yes* answer (the arm is weak). This is the vivaxis weak position. You will then find the exact direction by minimizing the degrees of rotation (until now 45°) and retesting until you find the specific direction in which the patient tests weakest.

Treatment of Vivaxis

With the patient continuing to hold the arm out in that exact position, like an antenna, you will then tap the head and sternum while the patient takes two full breath cycles.

Retest to make sure it is corrected Then move on and try the rest of the compass circle.

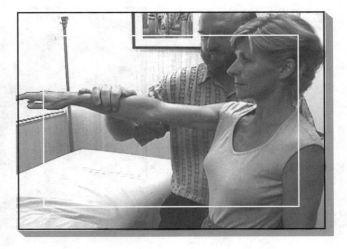

The Basic Cortices

Testing the Basic Cortices

- Run your hand lightly over the head of the patient just brushing the scalp as much as the hair will allow. This action should run from the front of the forehead, right over the head, to the base of the skull.

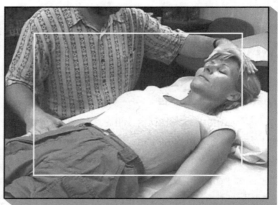

Running the cortices

- When you have done this, ask the body, *"Is there a problem with cortices?"* If the answer is *yes* (weak) then proceed with the treatment.

Treating the Cortices

- Place your hand on the patient's head at the base of the skull and upper neck. While you hold that position, tap the head and sternum, alternating for a full breath cycle.

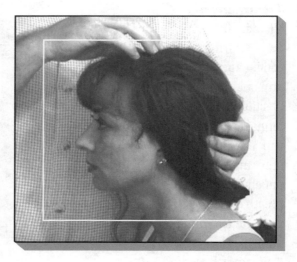

Tapping out the cortices

- Now move your hand up onto the head to the position next to the one you just did. (You are going to systematically cover the whole head.) In the new position, tap out the head and sternum alternating for a full breath.

148

- This procedure is repeated until you have covered the whole mid-line of the head. It usually takes four positions, although small hands on a big head may take five.
- You now need to cover the side of the head. Have the patient put one hand along the side of the head while you put your hand on the other side. Use your free hand to tap head and sternum, again while the patient takes a full breath.

Hydration

Testing Hydration
- Soak a tissue or cotton bud in some clean water.
- Place the wet tissue to the patient's navel or, if that is hard to get at because of clothing, you can place it over the thymus gland on the sternum.
- You then ask, "Is there a hydration problem?" If the answer is *yes* (weak) then the patient needs treatment.

Treating Hydration
- Leave the wet tissue in the navel and have your patient place their hands on the sides of their head so that the hands extend from the sphenoid bone (the temples) along to the area above the ears.

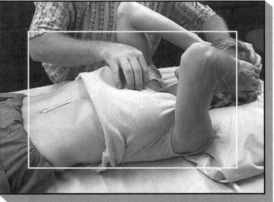

Treating hydration

- *You will then treat the cortices as you did in the cortex treatment.*
- Place your hand on the patient's head at the base of the skull and upper neck. While you hold that position, tap the head and sternum alternating for a full breath cycle.

- Now move your hand up onto the head to the position next to the one you just did. (You are going to systematically cover the whole head.) In the new position, tap out the head and sternum alternating for a full breath.
- This procedure is repeated until you have covered the whole mid-line of the head. It usually takes four positions although small hands on a big head may take five. (You do not need to do the sides of the head as you did with the basic cortices because they are already covered by the patient's hands.)

Scars and Skin Blockages

Testing for Scars and Skin Blockages

- To test to see if a scar is causing problems you need to challenge (poke) the scar while you muscle test. This poke is firm but not strong enough to cause discomfort.
- You ask, *"Is there a problem with this scar?"* If the answer is *yes* then the scar should be treated.

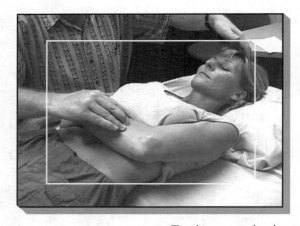

Treating scars and moles

Treatment for Scars and Skin Blockages

To treat the scar you continue to challenge (poke) the scar repeatedly while you tap out the head and sternum and you ask the patient to breathe deeply for two full breath cycles.

Retest

You should then retest the scar to confirm that the correction is successful.

Treating the Organs

- Ask, "Is balancing the organs the priority?" If the answer is *yes*, go on to step two. If the answer is *no*, leave the organs alone and go on to the next section.

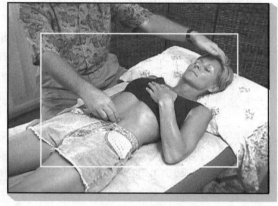

Linking the small intestine to the heart

- Now systematically place your hands on the organ reflex points illustrated in the photos. Start with the lungs and say, "Is the lung a priority?" If *yes*, go to step 3. If *no*, go to the next organ (heart) and ask if it is the priority. Keep going until you find the priority organ. My suggested order is Lungs, Heart, Liver, Gall Bladder, Stomach, Pancreas, Small Intestines, Colon, Bladder, Kidneys.

- Have the patient contact the priority organ (in this case, lung) while you systematically go to each organ and ask if it is the correct link for the lung. For example, "Link to heart?" *no*; "Link to liver?" *no*; "Link to stomach?" *yes*. Once you have a *yes*, go to step 4.

- While the patient holds the first organ (in this case—the lung) and the practitioner holds the linked organ (stomach), tap out the head and sternum while the patient takes two full breaths.

- Maintain the contacts and retest to ensure that the problem is corrected. "Is this link now a problem?" *no*.

- You will now ask if there are any further links to the first organ. (In this case, the lungs.) If the answer is *yes*, you then find the next organ to link it to and treat is as before. If the answer is *no*, you start again at step 2 and find the next priority organ that needs to be linked to another organ.

Blood Chemistry

- You now ask "Is there a problem with blood chemistry?" If the answer is *yes*, go on to the next step. (If the answer is *no,* it means that even if there is a problem, the body is not prepared to treat it at the moment. It may be that the body wants a few hours or days to correct itself more from the earlier treatments. It may also simply mean that there are no problems in this area. (Healthy people do actually exist!)

- Take a Q-tip or small piece of tissue and rub it on the patient's gums to get a sample of saliva and traces of blood. This will provide you with the point of reference for the body. The Q-tip is placed on a high energy center of the body so that the innate wisdom can 'read' it. I suggest that the best place is in the navel (belly button). If that is hard to access because of clothing, the left ear or the sternum can be used. This saliva-soaked Q-tip now becomes the focus of information with which the innate wisdom gathers knowledge of what is going on specifically within the body.

- Ask (using your muscle test) what the priority problem is. For example, "Is there a virus? If *yes,* go to step three to treat the virus. If *no*, ask the next question. "Is there an infection?" If *yes*, treat the infection. If *no* ask further until you find what the body wants to treat.

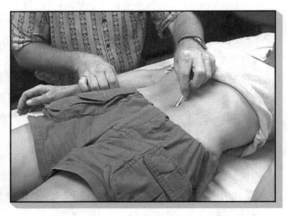

Testing saliva on tissue

Sample questions: "Is there a parasite?" "Is there an allergy?" "Is there a toxin?"

- Make sure you and the patient are aware of what you are treating (for example, virus) and have the patient place their hands on either side of their head. The hands will cover the temples to the upper half of their ears. This connects the limbic part of the brain to the treatment that is vital for results. (The reason for this is not covered in this book—just be happy with the clinical results!)

- While the patient keeps their hands on the sides of their heads you will then treat the cortices as you did in the cortex treatment. That is:
  1) Place your hand on the patient's head at the base of the skull and upper neck. While you hold that position, tap the head and sternum, alternating for a full breath cycle.
  2) Now move your hand up onto the head to the position next to the one you just did. (You are going to systematically cover the whole head.) In the new position, tap out the head and sternum alternating for a full breath.
  3) This procedure is repeated until you have covered the whole mid-line of the head. It usually takes four positions although small hands on a big head may take five. (You do not need to do the sides of the head as you did with the basic cortices since they are already covered by the patient's hands.)

Retest for Blood Chemistry

Now retest for the condition you treated (for example, virus) by asking, "Is there a virus?" If the answer is *no*, move on to the next question (infection, parasites, etc.).

Treating the Chakras

The treatment with BodyTalk is very simple. It follows the same pattern as with organs.

- We have to touch the focus point of each of the chakras (see photos) starting from the base chakra and ask, "Is there a problem with this chakra?" If the answer is *yes*, go to step 2. If the answer is *no*, ask the next chakra.
- Have the patient touch that chakra and look for the chakra to which it has a link. For example, the sexual (2) chakra may have indicated first. The patient places her hands over the chakra while you ask for the link. Is it (3)? (solar plexus) If the answer is *yes*, go to step 3. If the answer is *no*, ask for the next link.
- The patient holds one chakra and the practitioner holds the other while

tapping out the head and sternum as the patient takes two full deep breaths.

- Check that link has been corrected by asking the link again.
- Ask if there are any further links to that chakra (in this case chakra (2), the sexual chakra.) If the answer is *yes*, find the new link to be treated as in step 3. If the answer is *no,* move on to the next chakra, and so on until you have corrected all the links the innate wisdom requires.

At this stage you are at the end of your knowledge of BodyTalk, but it does not necessarily end there. Once you have completed the chakras, the general balance of the body may have shifted considerably to accommodate the changes.

At this stage in the treatment you will then ask, "Is there any further treatment today?" If the answer is *yes,* it means that the innate wisdom now wants you to go back and redo some of the earlier treatments so that it can 'fine tune' the system.

In this case you begin again, from the beginning, and see what comes up. Often it may just want you to balance two organs or treat another allergy.

If the answer to the question, "Is there any further treatment today?" was *no,* your treatment is finished.

You may then ask if the patient needs further treatment in the future. If the answer is *yes*, then you will need to find out when. The procedure is to ask for a time. For example, "Treat in less than a week?" If *yes*, then ask by the day. One day? Two days? Three days? etc.

If the answer was *no*, then ask by the week. One week? Two weeks? Three weeks? etc.

By this stage you will have given the type of treatment your body could only dream of receiving until now. You have asked its innate wisdom what to treat, in what order, and when to treat it. You have increased the total communication within the body so it can do its job better. You have linked the parts so they can once again function as a synchronized whole. You have not actually treated anyone yourself. The body will treat itself. You have acted as an impartial, objective facilitator for the bodymind lucky enough to find you and be balanced by BodyTalk.

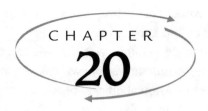

CHAPTER

20

Conclusion

THIS BOOK HAS ONLY SCRATCHED THE SURFACE OF THE BODYTALK SYSTEM. I sincerely hope that it will inspire you to try The BodyTalk System™ on your friends or patients and discover its magic.

Should you now feel a desire to have a BodyTalk treatment yourself then I would suggest you look at the directory of BodyTalk practitioners on the web site for the International BodyTalk Association (IBA), **www.bodytalksystem.com** . You can also look at our personal web site, which covers the other health care and personal growth tools my wife and I teach: **www.parama.com**.

If you want to go further than that, you will find a list of BodyTalk instructors on the same web site. Learning BodyTalk is very rewarding and the instructors trained and sanctioned by me through the IBA are highly qualified.

If you do not have internet access then I suggest you contact us in Florida, USA at **1-941-378-3341** so we can send you an IBA membership list.

The BodyTalk protocol that is taught in Modules 1 and 2 is the basis of the system. If that protocol is followed, the results will flow, even for a lay person. If you have other training, however, the protocol allows for this by having different sections that each skill can tap into. This difference being that each practitioner, no matter what their background, will still go through the basic treatments to satisfy the general balancing of the bodymind. Then, as you come to your specialty area, the innate wisdom of the body will lead you into your specialty so that it can take advantage of that knowledge.

For example, if you are a chiropractor, you will find that when you arrive at the section on the spine, the innate wisdom will ask you to balance the spine with BodyTalk and then let you know if quicker results will be obtained with adjustments. It will tell you what to adjust and *in what sequence*! The order in which you adjust the spine is vital for fast and lasting results.

In another example, acupuncturists will come to the section on meridians and find that the innate wisdom may ask them to use specific acupuncture points. Again, there is a protocol of point selection and sequencing of needle insertions that will greatly improve results.

Further, a psychologist will use her specialized training to be able to use the section on emotional treatments more effectively.

Naturopaths and medical practitioners can use the blood chemistry section to establish the need for supplements, herbs, or drugs. The key will be the ability to neutralize any harmful side effects and to establish exactly what dosage to give and at what frequency. The list goes on.

In the future, the IBA will be putting together video tapes and lectures on these specialty fields with Module 1 and 2 as a prerequisite. Within a few years there will be 'general practitioner' BodyTalk practitioners, lay practitioners helping friends and family with simple treatments, and specialist BodyTalk practitioners who will cover the tough cases relating to their field of expertise.

The BodyTalk System™ also lends itself very well to the future trend of multidisciplined clinics where practitioners from many different fields—conventional and alternative—share a clinic, enabling them to provide the best services for their patients. By having each participating practitioner trained in the BodyTalk protocol, there will be a foundation of common language and reference points for effective interdisciplinary cooperation. They will be able to let the patient's innate wisdom guide them to the right therapies, in right sequence, at the right time.

I am particularly looking forward to seeing nurses in hospitals trained in BodyTalk so they can maximize the patient's recovery time. By balancing the patient before surgery or therapy, the patient will respond much faster. Then, after the surgery, by treating the scars and rebalancing the body to the new energy dynamics created by the surgery, the patient will recover in a third of the time. Imagine the dramatic savings in health care costs for both the patients and communities.

One of the most exciting aspects of BodyTalk lies in total health care costs. The BodyTalk System™ is a low frequency treatment system. Although there are exceptions in very difficult cases, the average number of treatments required in BodyTalk is two to four initially. The patient then often needs to have monthly rebalancing for a few months to reestablish the new energy patterns into a lasting formula. In the USA the average treatment costs between $50.00 and $80.00. When you add up the sums, the savings are enormous!

Thank you for taking this journey into discovering BodyTalk with me. I have no doubt that you will hear a great deal more about BodyTalk in the future. I firmly believe that BodyTalk, or its equivalent under different names, will be a household word within ten years.

If you use the essential basic BodyTalk treatment as an adjunct to an existing health care modality, the results will speak for themselves. If you are a layperson who simply wishes to take a more active part in your family's health care, your lack of foundation in medical terminology is not a drawback. The beauty of The BodyTalk System™ is that it does not rely on the subjective diagnostic skills of a practitioner. Just trust in the body—it has all the answers and it has simply been waiting to be heard.

Dr. John Veltheim

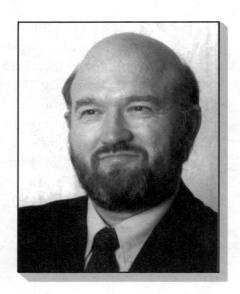

John is a chiropractor, traditional acupuncturist, philosopher, Reiki master and writer. He ran a very successful clinic in Brisbane, Australia, for 15 years. He was also the Principal of the Brisbane College of Acupuncture and Natural Therapies for five years. His extensive post graduate studies include applied kinesiology, bioenergetic therapy, osteopathy, sports medicine, counselling and comparative philosophy and theology.

John, with his wife Esther, has been lecturing on the international lecture circuit for seven years; teaching MindScape, Breakthrough, Reiki, philosophy, The BodyTalk System™, and life sciences. John teaches regularly in Australia, New Zealand, Hong Kong, Malta, England, Sweden, Switzerland and the United States. He founded The BodyTalk System™ and wrote the teaching manuals. He coauthored, with Esther, the book *Reiki: The Science, Metaphysics and Philosophy*, and has written a book on acupuncture and published many articles on a wide variety of modalities.

John and Esther also founded the *PaRama School of Philosophy and Life Sciences.*

PaRama and Dr. Veltheim can be contacted at;
5500 Bee Ridge Rd., Suite 103
Sarasota, Florida, 34233, USA
Fax (941) 342-8105
e-mail: **parama@home.com**
Web site: **www.parama.com**

For a list of BodyTalk practitioners, lecturers and workshop schedules:
IBA website: **www.bodytalksystem.com**